# Disc

MW01226200

## No warranties

The authors, publishers, trainers or contractors do not guarantee or warrant the quality, accuracy, completeness, timeliness, appropriateness or suitability of the information in this book. The information in this book is provided on an "as is" basis and the authors and publishers make no representations or warranties of any kind with respect to this information. This book may contain inaccuracies, typographical errors, or other errors.

## Liability disclaimer

The authors, publishers or any other parties involved in the creation and production of information in this book disclaim any responsibility and shall not be liable for any damages, claims, injuries, losses, liabilities, costs or obligations. This includes any direct, indirect, special, incidental or consequential damages whatsoever or howsoever caused.

## Health disclaimer

The intention of this book is to provide essential information for educational purposes only and that is not specific to you, the reader. The contents are intended to assist you in your personal wellness efforts. Nothing in this book should be taken as a diagnosis or personal advice, and must *not* be used in this manner. You should consult with your physician before beginning any exercise rehabilitation, weight loss or health care program. This book *should not* be used in place of a visit to a competent health-care professional. If you suspect you have a health-care problem, you should immediately contact a qualified health care professional for treatment. This book IS NOT giving you medical advice.

Exercise disclaimer

Exercise is not without its risks. Read that again. Any exercise program and all its movements may result in injury. Risks include but are not limited to: aggravation of a pre-existing condition, risk of injury, or adverse effect of over-exertion. Over-exertion can include muscle strain, abnormal blood pressure, fainting, disorders of heartbeat, heart attack or even death.

# Copyright

retrieval system, is forbidden without he express written permission of the author.

Although the authors and editors have made every effort to ensure the accuracy and completeness of information contained in this book, it is difficult to ensure that all of the information is accurate, and the possibility of error can never be completely eliminated. The authors and editors disclaim any liability or responsibility for injury or damage to persons or property that is incurred as a consequence, directly or indirectly, of the use and application of any of the contents of this book, as well as for any unintentional slights to any person or entity. See the Disclaimers for more details.

# Acknowledgements

I like to dedicate this book to my family, coworkers and all clients/patients of the past, present and future, and anyone who supported me along the way. Thank you for all that you have taught me and how you shaped me to the person I am today. I will forever be grateful. I hope this book will help everyone reach their physical goals.

I also like to make a special acknowledgement to Dennet Lee. You have taught and grew me to an unbelievable level of human being. You have pushed me to a level which I thought was impossible to get to. Without you, this book would not exist. Thank you.

# Table of Contents

- Types, Anatomy and Cause
- Frozen shoulder
- Labral tear of the shoulder
- Shoulder bursitis
- Shoulder separation
- Shoulder dislocation
- Shoulder blade pain
- Biceps tendon tear
- Treatments

## 6. Elbow, wrist & hand Injuries - pg. 118

- Golfer's elbow
- Tennis elbow
- Carpal tunnel syndrome
- Wrist and hand fracture (fifth metacarpal fracture)
- Finger fracture
- Treatments

## 7. Lower back & Hip Injuries - pg. 151

- Causes & symptoms; Case about gluteus medius
- Lower cross syndrome (lower back pain)
- Middle back pain
- Hip fracture
- Hip flexor strain
- Snapping hip syndrome
- SLAP tear (Labrum tear)
- SI joint pain

## 8. Leg & Knee Injuries - pg. 215

- Knee science and kinetic chain
- Sciatica (piriformis syndrome)
- Jumper's knee (patellar tendon injury)
- Strained hamstrings
- Torn meniscus
- Torn ACL and/or PCL (anterior cruciate ligament & posterior cruciate ligament)

- Shin splints

- Ankle sprain
- Achilles tendon rupture
- Plantar fasciitis
- High ankle sprain

# **0:** Introduction: What is this book?

What are you doing here? Well obviously you are here to obtain additional information regarding physical health, strength and everlasting well-being. You could be here because you suffered an injury, or have friends/family who suffered an injury, or you're in the healthcare field looking to add knowledge and depth in your practice.

This is a book on EXERCISE THERAPY; or if you are IN the field it is referred to as ACTIVE REHABILITATION (most likely shortened to rehab). Both of these are the same idea. It's defined as "a regimen of physical activities designed and prescribed to patients to recover from diseases and any conditions that disturb their movement and/or activities of daily life".

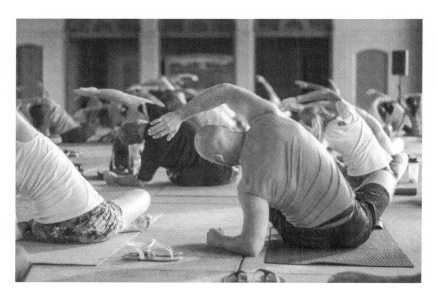

*Mahapatra (2019).*

My personal definition is "a specifically tailored exercise program prescribed to a patient that targets movement deficiencies and limited strength & mobility to decrease pain symptoms, increase quality of life and improve performance".

The goal of exercise therapy can be achieved in countless number of ways. Some include strength training, mobility instruction, brain rewiring, gait training, etc. The goal remains the same but the choice of route is in your hands. The realm of this field is so big that you can never run out of resources. Dig deep and get CREATIVE.

Usually, exercise therapy is often performed and guided with a registered kinesiologist. Kinesiology is simply a study of human movement that addresses physiological, biomechanical and psychological principles. Therefore, as a patient, you are working with someone with a special set of skills, who will help you cope with pain and will guide you towards recovery and strength. It doesn't get better than that!

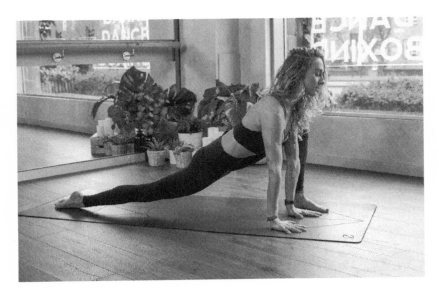

*Form (2019).*

I get this question quite frequently: is a kinesiologist and personal trainer the same? NO, they are NOT the same! In fact there are major differences. Kinesiology is SCIENTIFIC. Personal training is not as scientific. Kinesiology is its own recognized field of study. It has research departments devoted to further the knowledge of human movement. You must go through a four or five year post-secondary degree program to become a kinesiologist. There is no degree in personal training. Personal trainers may get certified through weekend courses or workshops. In short: kinesiology is medical, personal training is not.

With all that said, there is a significant overlap with the prescription below. You will see progressions and regressions of exercises that will combine the two professions. Exercise prescriptions will almost always begin with "rehab" type training which will then progress into higher intensity exercise. At the end of the program it will look a lot like a personal training session with exercises designed to improve functional strength. And that is the MAIN IDEA of this book. It is to bridge the gap between rehabilitation and functional strength training. Most rehabilitation program stop at where the pain has subsided, but the patient has not improved their strength. Gains are plateaued and chances of re-injury are high. The point here is to push past the rehab exercises and strength train functionally so that patients can go back to everyday living PAIN-FREE and STRONG.

# 1. How to use this book

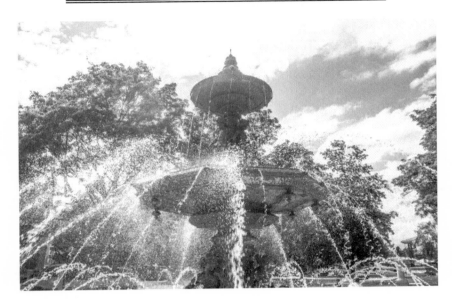

*Jones (2015).*

The above picture is the fountain of youth (not really).

If there was a fountain of youth and if you drank from it you would become pain-free forever, would you drink from it? If it gave you the ability to "move and FEEL like you're young again", would you drink from it?

This fountain supposedly restores the youth of anyone who drinks or bathes in its waters. The tales of such a fountain have been recounted across the world for thousands of years, appearing in writings by Herodotus (5th century BC). Later in 1513, Ponce de Leon (a Spanish explorer) was told by Native Americans that the Fountain of Youth could restore youth to anyone.

Unfortunately, in 2019 AD this fountain of youth does not exist (or at least I do not know of). The good news is that in this modern age we not have to go through wars, diseases or famine. These three alone would have killed off many of our ancestors and we would be constantly looking for ways to combat these attackers. It wouldn't be pain we would be concerned about; it would be straight death. But in modern society, we are free from those concerns.

This book is giving you the direct flight to the fountain of youth. It is going to give you the tools you need to restore your earlier life and make it EVERLASTING. If you are injured, also known as "physically sick", I am giving you the MEDICINE to heal your body. There is no overdose limit to this type of medicine. I highly encourage you to take this medicine as often as you can.

## Impact of Technology

In the modern world we live in, technology impacts our entire humankind both positively and negatively. At a medical level, technology has a tremendous role in treating patients more effectively and efficiently as ever. Medicine has developed into an ever perpetuating field that can accomplish feats that were deemed impossible in the past. Diseases, viruses and bacteria are combatted at an incredible rate due to advancement of technology.

For non-medical professionals, efficiency is highly enhanced because communication has improved so much. Before was mail, then e-mail came along, now we are able to view the other person and environment with full color and sound in real-time. How amazing is that! There is no longer any delays with communicating, which is why tasks are able to be completed at so efficiently.

So what is negative about technology? Well with technology, humans physically do less in order to achieve the same outcome. For example, instead of walking up to the television to turn it on or adjust the volume, we have a remote to do all these functions at the comfort of our sofa. Instead of walking to the restaurant to get our take-out, we have special delivery services to get us our food from a click at our computer. We have all these at our disposal without doing or moving a lot. And this is where problems occur. There is a saying, "sitting is the new smoking". I completely, 100% agree with this saying. The impact of technology has humans sitting more than ever and will increase as time goes on. Eventually this will (or has already) become toxic. Who knows? Maybe soon we will need technology to remove our technology.

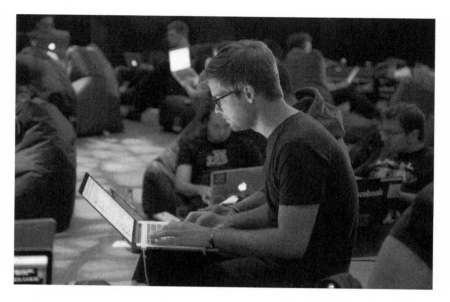

*Kotliarsky (2017).*

More specifically, the additions of the smartphone or iPads have added additional burdens onto our physical well-being. With phones and tablets, our necks are in flexion for a large period of our day - putting a strain on our spine. Sitting for prolonged periods of time caves our shoulders forward due to gravity and causes pain in our shoulders and upper back. Inactivity even causes an increase in body fat, blood pressure and cholesterol. This can even lead to obesity or even a stroke. These are devastating effects of modern day technology.

But FEAR NOT! Although technology will only get more advanced and more convenient, there IS fix to the consequences. This is the medicine I mentioned earlier. Movement. Exercise. And rehab - if you have any injuries or strains. TAKE YOUR MEDICINE!

The medicine I'm giving you is highly accessible and can be performed by individuals of all levels from highly competitive athlete to someone who has never exercised before. And this method will be incredibly cost effective compared to a cortisol shot or any other surgical method. You put in a very little expense, perhaps a pair of supportive running shoes and a set of gym clothes, and you get a very high quality return. Take-away point: by taking a little of this "medicine" per day, you can setback numerous debilitating effects of inactivity and technology.

# **2.** The SYSTEM

What you will learn in this book is an extensive system built for the injured individual, someone who experiences "strain" from daily activities, or someone who is looking to start being active. The toughest part, whether it be rehabilitation or fitness, it getting started. I understand. It's a hard push. It's an uphill battle for most if not all of the journey. But every time you face a challenge or don't want to do the exercises, remind yourself of what benefits it will bring to you. Do you want to be pain-free? Do you want to be stronger? Do you want to feel young again?

The key here is to have faith. You simply just need to jump in. Things will figure itself out. Don't second guess yourself or do excessive research. You will end up convincing yourself out of it. Trust the system. Let's go!

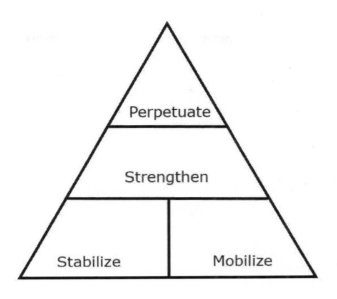

## 1.) **FOUNDATION = STABILITY + MOBILITY**

Begin at the bottom. This is where foundation and basics are built. The make-up of human movement revolves around **stability** and **mobility**; the ability to resist movement and to produce movement. Take walking as an example. The swinging leg is responsible for translating the leg around the hip joint (mobility), preparing for the next step and moving the body forward. At the same time the supporting leg is responsible for keeping the hips and trunk stable (stability) as the swinging leg makes its movement. Both go hand-in-hand. The body, or that region, will crumble if the foundation don't cooperate well with each other.

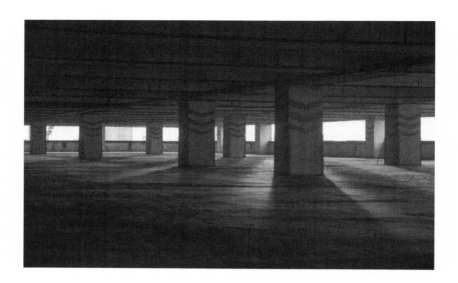

*Blicke (2017).*

- Without mobility, the swinging leg would have very inefficient movement so you wouldn't be able to step very far. Of course, strength makes up a significant part in the swinging leg and stepping. It is the movement through the joint which is the focus at this stage of rehab - not the absolute strength.
- Let's not confuse the difference between flexibility and mobility here. **Flexibility** is the ability of a muscle to lengthen. **Mobility** is the ability of a joint to move through a range of motion actively or with tension. At this stage of rehab we are focusing on moving in the joint space actively using our muscles. Instead of statically holding a stretch, we are engaging the proper muscle to guide the joint through its allocated range-of-motion.

- **Stability** is the body's ability to resist a movement. Without stability, using walking as an example, our supporting leg would crumble along with our trunk. Along with movement in other areas of our body, keeping stable in other areas is critical. Think isolations, where we are activating muscles but not actually moving through the joint.

**\*\*\* How hard/intense should I be training? \*\*\***

This is a "ask yourself" question. How are your pain levels when you are doing the foundation exercises?

I often instruct patients to train at an intensity of a pain threshold of 30% or 3/10 with 10 being extreme pain. At this threshold a slight pain or discomfort should be felt but not so intense that it causes you to cringe your face or curl your toes. The intensity to be training at should challenge your body and the proper muscles but not to the point where you need to give up. You need to push, but not too much

The sensation felt should be a "muscle burning" feeling, and you will be able to differentiate between a "good" pain and the "bad" pain. If you feel something like "bone on bone" or simply just wrenching pain, either take a break or regress the exercise to a less-intense variation.

At the end of your training session you should feel "generally better" and a little tired. The exercises prescribed allows you to target the problematic area without over exacerbating the symptoms too much (only if you don't progress too fast.

## 2.) **STRENGTHEN**

Once you have significant foundation in place and most pain symptoms have been managed, you may proceed into strengthening. With musculoskeletal injures, the body acts like a balance-scale. With trauma, one side of the scale "overloaded" and the other isn't loaded at all - making this scale imbalanced. The point of rehab is to balance the scale out so no part is compensating for any other parts. At this phase we are targeting key muscles to target imbalances of the injured areas. Don't think of squats or push-ups. Think of more low-intensity, single-joint exercises that target small muscle groups.

In this phase, it is important to note that it is very important to be aware of which muscle you are targeting. Make the mind-to-muscle connection as you are performing these movements. However, you may not necessarily feel a "burn" during these exercises. Jst feel the muscles "working" and doing what they're supposed to. Remember it is not a high-intensity workout. This is rehab.

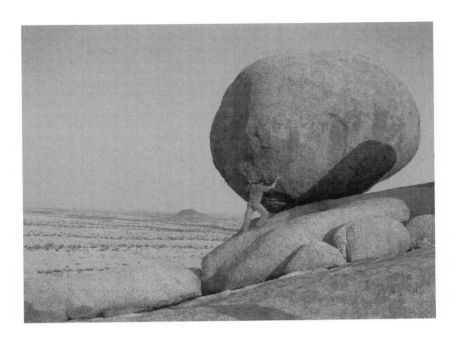

*Vicky Sim (2017).*

### 3.) **PERPETUATE**

You have arrived at the part where ANTI-AGING and living PAIN-FREE forever come into play. You have successfully recovered, regained your range-of-motion, most of your symptoms are managed and have increased in overall strength. But is that the end? Do we stop here and carry on with life? Definitely not! Patients I have previously treated who have successfully recovered that do not maintain their strength and mobility, experience a RELAPSE of symptoms. It comes back to haunt you if you don't maintain it!

It is absolutely crucial that individuals keep up with a maintenance program. Perpetual is defined as "never ending or changing". Progress must be maintained in order for strength, stability and mobility to be kept on par and GREAT HEALTH to be "never ending or changing".

This is the stage where we **bridge the gap between rehab and strength training**. The exercises and programming here will look a lot like the training you see in a personal training class. Weights and machines will be used. You will also see high-intensity movements such as plyometric or jumping movements. The intensity is definitely higher at this stage because we have built our body in terms of mobility and stability to control this intensity. And as always, ask yourself how it feels and how it's supposed to feel to gauge a proper intensity.

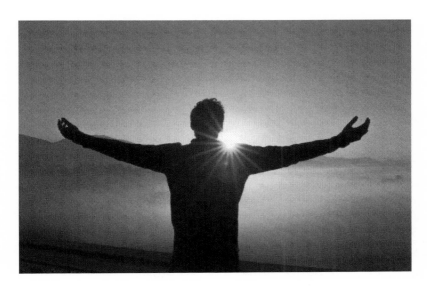

*Durant (2017).*

## 4.) **STAPLE STRETCHES**

This component encompasses the entire system. At the end of every section of a region, you will find a list of stretches. Regardless of which injury you have, it is highly recommended that you complete those stretches after every rehab/training session. Unless you are a hyper-flexible individual, which most of the population is not, stretching is a must. If an area has experienced recent acute trauma, it is recommended to rest it and keep it non-active. During the resting period, range-of-motion of the affected region and surrounding muscle decreases. This causes even more of an imbalance in the body. Training for stability and mobility can be post-pone for a later time, but keeping **flexibility** is highly recommended. Here we are talking about the ability of a muscle to lengthen.

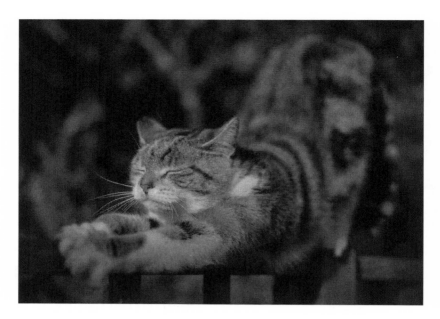

*Tasi (2017).*

## When to progress?

When do you know it is time to move onto the next stage in your training? When do you know you are READY to increase the intensity and/or volume to your training?

Well there is never a definite answer. It all depends on how you feel on your current progress. You need to judge based on your subjective observations and how comfortable you are with the prescribed movements.

Is your pain level kept at 30% or below during all exercises? Could you finish all the exercises within a reasonable time frame? Are all exercises done with high quality of movement with good posture and full range-of-movement?

If all these questions can be answered with full confidence, you can progress. You will know when you can move up. Please keep in mind that the next level exercises will challenge your body and mind even further. If you feel that the intensity is too much for your symptoms, there is no shame in regressing back to the previous level.

## **2.** Mindset and Lifestyle change

When you get injured, your body goes through numerous biomechanical, physiological and biochemical changes. So what should we do?

Life goes on. Your body does what it can do keep you functioning. One side compensates to balance out the other. The bottom side works harder to support the top. Your body makes it all work by altering its natural movement to accommodate new changes. However, because this new "program" is no longer natural, surrounding muscles and connective tissues are no stressed. This becomes a downward spiral if you DO NOT TAKE CARE OF YOUR BODY. The longer you leave it, the harder it becomes to fix the issue. I highly urge you to take action IMMEDIATELY.

Before we dive in detail about musculoskeletal solutions, I need to emphasize another tool in our arsenal for a maximum recovery - your MIND.

**Mindset**

Yes, I understand you are in pain. I understand you don't want to move because you are afraid of experiencing pain or re-aggravating your symptoms. I understand you are frustrated because you wish you weren't injured and you are missing out on life.

I completely understand. But believe it or not, the biggest limitation to a maximum recovery – is you. Well, specifically, it's your brain. Your mindset is your biggest mental block. Pain is created in the brain so if you "rewire" how you think you can get over this wall.

Below are some tools that are your keys to overcome any mental block during this rehab process.

1.) Awareness

- Being aware of incoming thoughts and learning how to RE-DIRECT them is absolutely critical. If you experience pain (which is understandable), stop, acknowledge it, and convert it to a healthy thought. This is difficult in the beginning but as this becomes routine, you can successfully re-wire your brain to translate what pain really is.
- Take this thought: "this really hurts! I need to stop and rest for a while". Now translate it to: "this really hurts, but I am able to take a break and slowly work my way back into it because I know it's good for me".

2.) Reframing thoughts

- Being able to turn unhealthy thoughts into constructive one is an even harder task. Once you are able to do it, you will see an entire lifestyle change. Remember, it is okay to have negative thought but it's crucial that you catch yourself and immediately reframe it to a positive one.

- Take this thought: "I'm going to be stuck with this pain forever". Now translate it to: "This hurts a lot right now but it's not permanent because I will recover".

3.) Use a Mantra

- A mantra is a few words you can say to yourself to calm the situation or re-gather yourself when things get tough. These words need to be powerful enough to alleviate any stress on the individual.
- Strong words in pain management are: *Release, relax, open, breathe, sink* or *slow.*

# 3. WHY does this all matter?

This section is for you to understand how this will all come together on a grand scheme of things. Our bodies go through different phases of healing depending on the trauma. Some musculoskeletal injuries may have a different timeline, while others may have many phases.

When you injure your body it undergoes biomechanical, physiological and biochemical changes. Injuries can stress your tissues and can even alter your walking pattern. Furthermore, injuries can cause micro-tears in the tissues, pinch your nerves and can compromise the cardiovascular system. These effects are broken down into more specific symptoms below.

| Micro-tears in tissues | Pinching in nerves | Compromised cardiovascular system |
|---|---|---|
| o Increased pain | o Increased pain | o Slower healing |
| o Increased tissue damage | o Decreased strength | o Decreased oxygen |
| o Increased inflammation | o Reduced nerve function | o Increased scar tissue formation |

**So how do tissues build themselves back up?**

Generally, tissues will go through three phases.

28

## 1. Acute inflammatory phase

This first phase occurs within the first 24 – 48 hours of injury and you will often experience pain and swelling in the injured area. Early in this phase, it is recommended that you use the P.R.I.C.E. protocol; which stands for protection, rest, ice, compression and elevation. This will help with pain management and swelling.

It is acceptable, if required, to take over-the-counter anti-inflammatory or pain medication to manage pain symptoms. It is best to stick to these medications within 72 hours of injury. If taken after, they could have a negative effect on the healing process.

Take away point: rest and protection is most important at this stage.

## 2. Regenerative or Repair phase

In this second phase, the body begins to repair the damaged tissues. Here the inflammation will have gone down and new collagen is being laid down. This also reduces the need of your body to protect your injury as new tissue begins to mature and strengthen. But it still needs to be protected; just not as much.

This is phase is where active rehabilitation and exercise therapy come into play. We can begin low-intensity movements in order to move the new tissues. Movement, in a pain-managed state, is crucial at this time. It will allow nutrients to flow into the injured area and allows wastes to leave. It is KEY to begin getting some motion into the injured area at the end of the acute inflammatory phase. This will accelerate the recovery process.

More importantly, without movement the tissue that is laid will be laid in a more random pattern, rather than in a specific direction that benefits the joint. This will ultimately lead to the development of unbalanced tissues, further complications or even increased chance of re-injury.

### 3. Remodeling phase

This last phase can last up to 12 months. With proper exercise prescription and execution, collagen fibres can increase in size, diameter and strength. As you progress your strengthening program the injured area will feel closer and closer to what it was before. But you must NOT stop. Healing is a continuum and needs to be kept as sustainable and consistent as possible. Without the correct exercises, the possibility of re-injury is high. Lack of exercise can result in decreased oxygen delivery to soft tissues, increased scar tissue formation and prevention from full recovery.

Strength training after injury is often misapplied in many aspects. Quality strength training integrates neuromuscular control, proper body mechanics, postural improvement and core strength. With that said, starting strength training too soon can also be detrimental in our recovery. We must first establish the foundation, such as stability and mobility, before beginning strength training.

## But WHY?

Because of SCIENCE! It is scientifically proven that active rehabilitation or simply just staying active will greatly decrease your pain symptoms and/or decrease the number of painful episodes in the future. I know it is way easier to go to a therapy session, lie down and let the therapist work on you (RMT or a physiotherapist). While these are amazing treatment methods, they must be done in CONJUNCTION with exercise. This is to improve muscular strength and endurance, as well as functional mobility. You must put in the work in order to optimize the treatment effect and relief, and to make permanent POSITIVE changes. Take-away point: TAKE ACTION NOW.

# **4.** Neck Pain Injuries

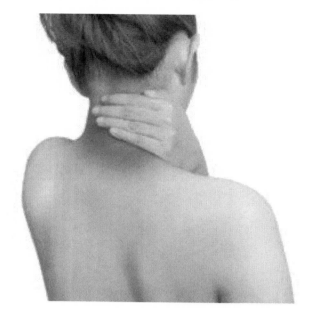

*Upper cervical chiropractic of Monmouth (2019)*

## Causes & Symptoms

Injuries to the neck can be minor or serious depending how what exactly happened and how severe it was. Think about it for a second. Your head is 10+ pounds and is attached by a smaller structure to your body. Then add a violent snap back and forth. This is a symptom to whiplash injuries in motor vehicle accidents and sporting injuries. When the head experiences a rapid back-and-fourth movement it is almost like the cracking of a whip.

A number of injuries occur in the neck area such as spasms, strain or even fractures. Patients will usually feel pain, stiffness, and even shooting pain down the arm. Depending on if there are concussions, patients may experience headaches, dizziness or nausea. Initially all these injuries are treated traditionally with heat, ice, physical therapy or even with muscle relaxants. As pain symptoms subside, individuals may begin integrating exercises to begin rehab.

Postural Awareness

The ability to know and feel how you are standing or sitting is incredibly important to recovery. As we know, our head is 10+ pounds. If you load it incorrectly onto your trunk, other muscles will compensate and ultimately alter the way your upper body is supposed to function.

- Muscles will overload; making key muscle groups working harder than necessary.
- Increased stress on the cervical spine; this area must work excessively to support the head.
- Bad head posture leads to a rounded back which may lead to more pain in the upper back.

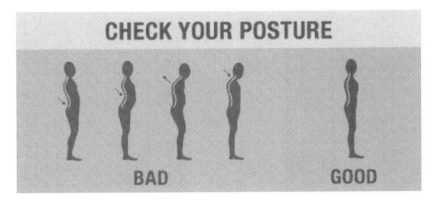

*Adelaide West Physiotherapy and Pilates Classes (2018).*

Here is a quick checklist for your current posture:

- ○ Chin up, head pushed back.
- ○ Shoulders rolled back AND down.
- ○ Very slight forward arch in the lower back.
- ○ Hips align with ankles.
- ○ Stand as tall as you can.

All these factors need to come together as a whole for what is considered "good posture". The sooner you can integrate this into your lifestyle, the sooner your body will re-wire what normal function is supposed to be. Remember this needs to be kept long-term for effects to be permanent.

**Don't be like this guy.**

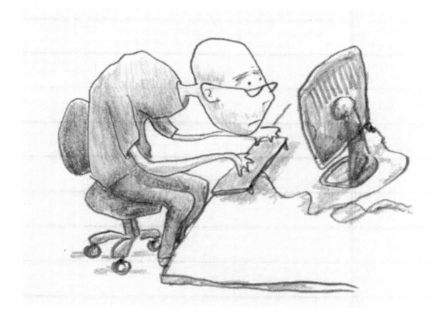

*Jockers (2014).*

## UPPER CROSS SYNDROME

So why does all of this matter?

Because of upper cross syndrome. Simply put it is a compensation of one muscle group when the other becomes weak or non-functioning. Take our balance scale as an example again. One side becomes overloaded and overworked while the other side is loaded less and eventually becomes stagnant. Here, our shoulders, neck and chest muscles become overloaded - while our neck flexors and upper back are functioning less than normal. The symptoms commonly caused are neck pain, headaches, chest tightness and other upper body discomfort. This syndrome isn't necessarily death-related or serious but the longer it is left untreated the more serious it becomes.

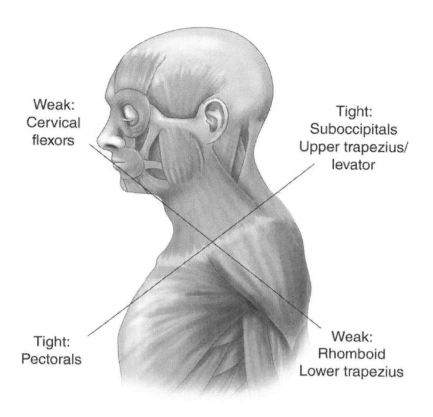

Weak:
Cervical
flexors

Tight:
Suboccipitals
Upper trapezius/
levator

Tight:
Pectorals

Weak:
Rhomboid
Lower trapezius

*Alpha Spine Center (2019).*

Let's take a look at the above diagram. The main concept is simple: strengthen those that are weak; stretch and mobilize those that are tight. There is countless number of ways to strengthen and stretch these muscles. Find the method that works best for you.

## Whiplash Injury

One of the more common injury: the whiplash. This commonly occurs to athlete with high-intensity sports;

however, it can also happen to people on a regular daily living basis. Most commonly, it is due to a car accident. A sudden trauma, or change of direction of the head, can cause a whiplash. This is a neck injury the results from a rapid hyperextension of the neck then thrown quickly into flexion.

A whiplash can cause a variety of symptoms including neck and shoulder pain, headaches, dizziness and fatigue, and vision problems. It is highly recommended that you see your doctor about this. In the acute stages, the doctor may prescribe some pain-killers and muscle relaxant. Once we are past the initial trauma and pain stage, we can begin treating it with exercise therapy.

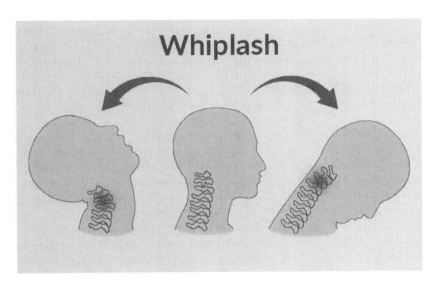

*pt Health (2018).*

Herniated Disc

This occurs when the soft, rubbery part between the bony structures is pushed out of position and presses on a nerve root. This usually happens when there is a rip in the outer fibres of the disc and can happen by a sudden or a repeated force.

Patients will generally complain of "burning", "electric shock" or "shooting pain" down the arm or leg. They may also report or demonstrate weakness or limited range-of-motion. Usually it would not feel "right" so as mentioned before your best bet is to see a doctor for a full physical examination and an X-ray. Almost always, active rehabilitation will not occur until at least the some type of physical therapy treatment and rest.

Sports related injuries and "tweaks"

Your neck is essentially a connection between your head and the rest of your body. They come in different shapes and sizes; some are wide and some are narrower. Regardless of how they are shaped, your neck has a very important job. It has to be flexible enough to move but it has to be strong enough to withstand any type of impact or sudden movement.

The reason why sports can cause a high number of neck injury is because of its unpredictable nature. Let's take ice hockey for example. Every time a player is on the ice, his head is essential on a "swivel". He is always turning his head; locating the puck, looking out for open ice and other players. This motion, with the weight of the helmet, already puts a strain on the supporting neck muscles. In ADDITION, depending on the level of play there may be impact in the sport. He may need to take a hit, he may lose his balance and fall, or there may be bumped accidentally. All these factors take a toll on the neck.

The protocol is simple: get it checked out and use the P.R.I.C.E. protocol. If it is an acute injury, we do not want to take any chances as there can be a wide variety of factors that can influence this injury. Your doctor and/or physical therapists will make recommendations. When pain is managed, we start exercise therapy.

# Neck Strain

### Mobilize: Chin tucks: *2 sets, 10 repetitions*.

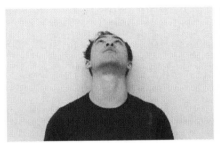 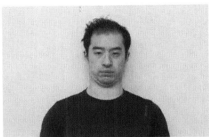

Pro-tip: Keep the back of your head on the wall at all times and press the chin downwards.

### Mobilize: Towel-supported extensions: *2 sets, 10 repetitions*.

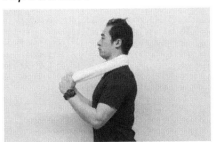 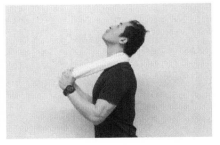

Pro-tip: The point of the towel is to support the weight of your head to restore the range.

## Mobilize: Quadraped neck rotations: *2 sets, 5 repetitions per side*.

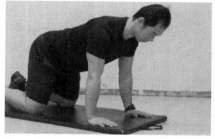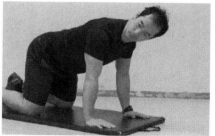

Pro-tip: Keep your shoulder blades engaged and rotate to tolerable pain.

## Stabilize: Scapular squeeze: *2 sets, 10 repetitions*.

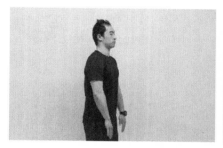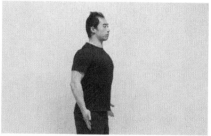

Pro-tip: As your squeeze your shoulder blades together, keep your shoulders down and your chin tucked in.

## Stabilize: Isometric neck flexion: *2 sets, 45 seconds*.

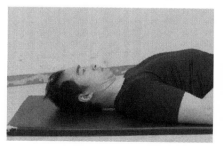

Pro-tip: Press your chin into your neck as hard as you can keeping your shoulders down.

### Stabilize: Tuck & Lift: *2 sets, 10 repetitions.*

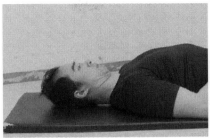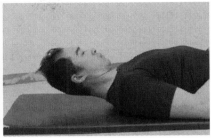

Pro-tip: You only need about two or three inches off the ground for one second of hold.

### Strengthen: Band rows: *4 sets, 15 repetitions.*

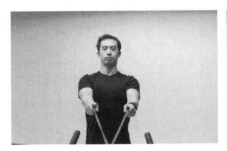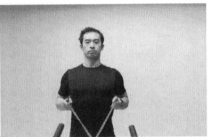

Pro-tip: Keep your shoulder blades down and back during the entire movement.

### Strengthen: Prone elbow lifts: *4 sets, 10 repetitions.*

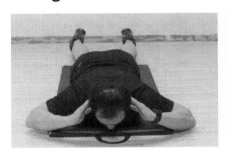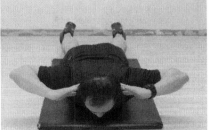

Pro-tip: Keep your shoulders down and lift the elbows as high as you can.

### Strengthen: Prone dowel pull-down: *4 sets, 10 repetitions.*

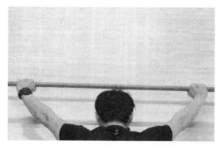 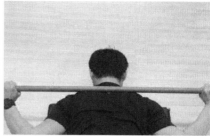

Pro-tip: Keep the movement controlled and straighten your arms at the end.

### Strengthen: Band external rotations: *4 sets, 15 repetitions.*

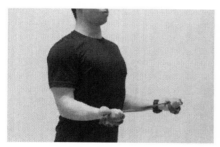 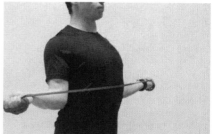

Pro-tip: Keep your elbows locked at 90 degrees during the entire movement.

## Perpetuate: Side bridges: *4 sets, 10 repetitions per side*.

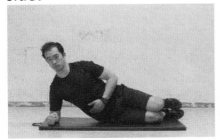 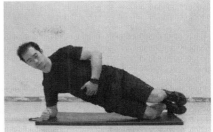

Pro-tip: Keep your shoulder blades "locked down" as you lift your hips up.

## Perpetuate: Underarm pull-downs: *4 sets, 15 repetitions.*

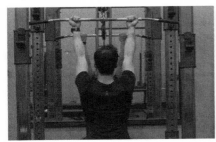 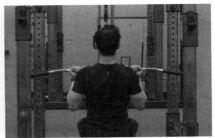

Pro-tip: Squeeze your shoulder blades together at the bottom of the movement.

**Perpetuate: Dumbbell shoulder press:** *4 sets, 10 repetitions.*

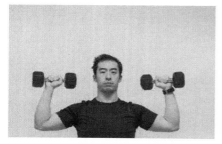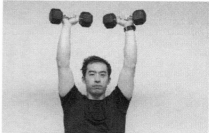

Pro-tip: Refrain from shrugging our shoulders at the top of the movement.

## Neck Spasms

**Mobilize: Foam roller thoracic extension:** *2 sets, 10 repetitions*.

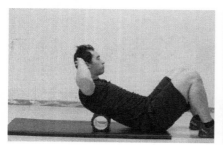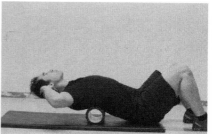

Pro-tip: The roller should stay right beneath the shoulder blades.

**Mobilize: Wall thoracic extension:** *2 sets, 10 repetitions.*

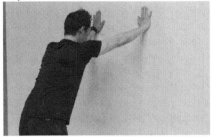 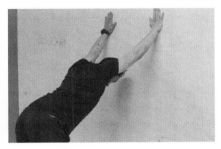

Pro-tip: You may slightly arch your trunk.

**Mobilize: Thoracic rotation:** *2 sets, 5 repetitions per side.*

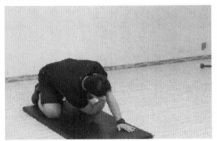 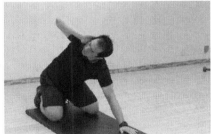

Pro-tip: Rock your hips back and sit on your heels as you rotate your trunk.

**Stabilize: Tuck, lift & curl:** *2 sets, 10 repetitions.*

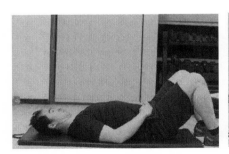 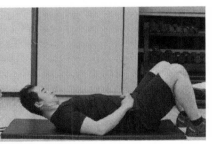

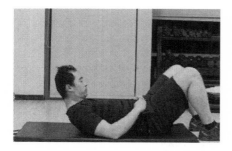

Pro-tip: Ensure that your chin is tucked in at all times during the head lift.

## Stabilize: Tuck, lift & side bend: *2 sets, 5 repetitions per side.*

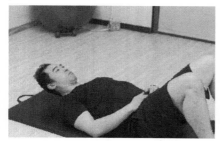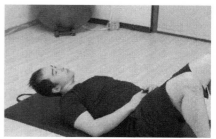

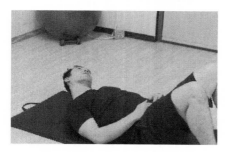

Pro-tip: Ensure that your chin is tucked throughout the entire movement.

**Stabilize: Tuck, lift & rotate:** *2 sets, 5 repetitions per side.*

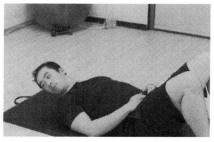

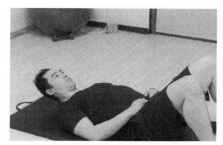

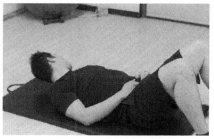

Pro-tip: Ensure that your chin is tucked throughout the entire movement. Lift your head to about two or three inches off the floor.

**Strengthen: Band Y & T:** *4 sets, 10 repetitions of Y then 10 of T.*

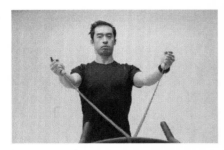
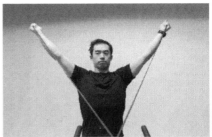
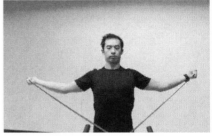

Pro-tip: Keep your shoulder blades back and down throughout both movements.

**Strengthen: Bent-over Ws & wing-spans:** *4 sets, 10 repetitions of each.*

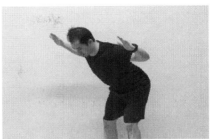

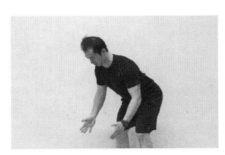

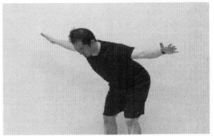

Pro-tip: Keep your chin tucked in and eyes down to ensure a straight spine.

**Strengthen: Prone single press-ups:** *4 sets, 10 repetitions per side.*

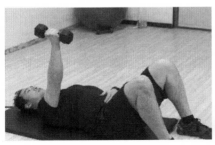

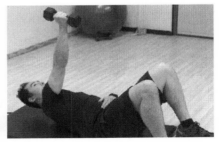

Pro-tip: This is a small movement and is targeting your rib cage muscles (serratus anterior).

## Strengthen: Serratus punches: *4 sets, 10 repetitions per side.*

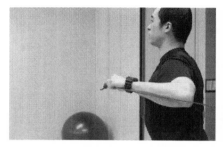 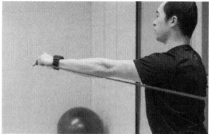

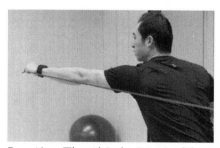

Pro-tip: The third picture (the reach) is the most important for targeting the proper muscle.

## Perpetuate: Bent over rows: *4 sets, 15 repetitions.*

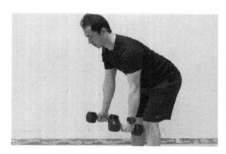 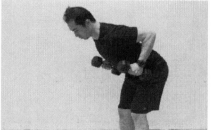

Pro-tip: Keep your elbows close to your body as you pull the weight into your body.

**Perpetuate: Dumbbell shoulder presses:** *4 sets, 15 repetitions.*

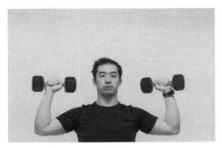 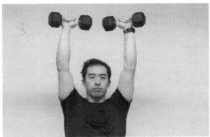

Pro-tip: Keep a tall posture as you push the weight upwards.

**Perpetuate: Overhead carries:** *3 sets, 45 seconds per arm.*

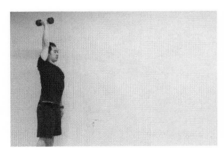 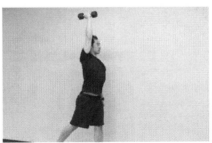

Pro-tip: Keep your shoulders from moving and coming up during the walk.

# Neck Nerve Pinch Injury

**Mobilize: Lacrosse ball smash:** *2 sets, 45 seconds on the affected side.*

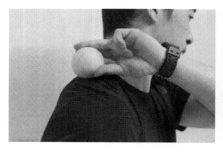 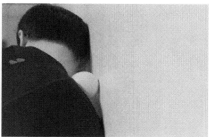

Pro-tip: Do not roll on my bony structures. Roll on any stiff/tight muscles.

**Mobilize: Ulnar nerve glide:** *2 sets, 10 repetitions on the affected side.*

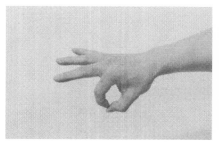 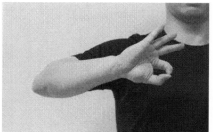

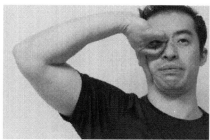

Pro-tip: The point is to point the pinky downwards. You may feel the numbness on the pinky side. Slowly work your way to the third picture.

**Mobilize: Median nerve glide:** *2 sets, 10 repetitions on the affected side.*

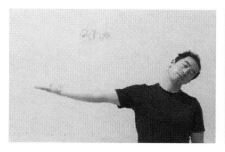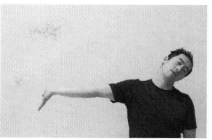

Pro-tip: You may feel a numbing "pulling" feeling on the top of the arm - that's the point.

**Mobilize: Radial nerve glide:** *2 sets, 10 repetitions on the affected side.*

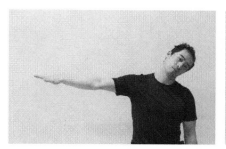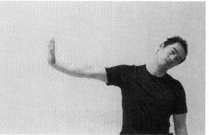

Pro-tip: If the stretch is too much, you may keep your head straight and work your way down.

**Stabilize: Wall angels:** *2 sets of 10 repetitions.*

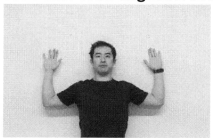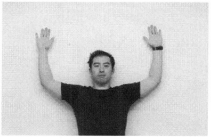

Pro-tip: Keep your elbows and wrist on the wall throughout the movement. It is a small movement.

### Stabilize: Tuck & extend: *2 sets of 10 repetitions.*

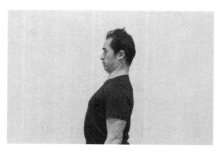 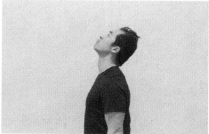

Pro-tip: Keep good posture during the movement and go as far as pain will allow it.

### Strengthen: Shoulder taps: *2 sets, 10 repetitions per side.*

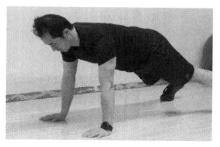 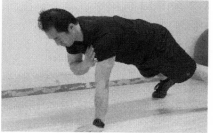

Pro-tip: Keep the supporting shoulder locked and stacked over the elbow and wrist.

**Strengthen: Elbow plank plus:** *4 sets, 10 repetitions.*

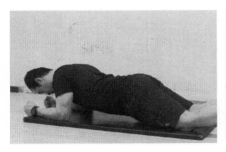 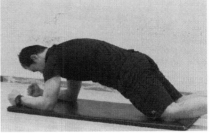

Pro-tip: The movement is at the shoulder blades - squeeze on the way down and release on the way up.

**Strengthen: Band Y overhead press:** *4 sets, 15 repetitions.*

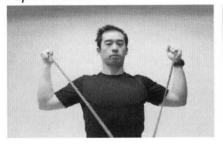 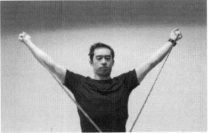

Pro-tip: Keep good posture and push your hands next to your body - not in front.

**Strengthen: Incline body butterflies:** *4 sets, 10 repetitions.*

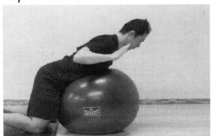 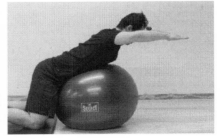

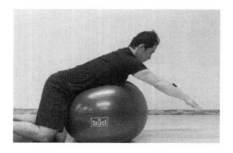

Pro-tip: Move in a circle going forward keeping shoulder blades squeeze - slow movement.

### Perpetuate: Cable face-pulls: *4 sets, 15 repetitions.*

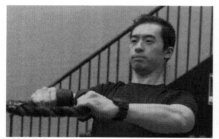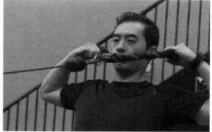

Pro-tip: Set the cable to chin level and pull with your elbows.

### Perpetuate: Front raises: *4 sets, 15 repetitions.*

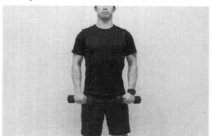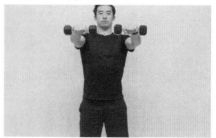

Pro-tip: Keep an upright posture and avoid any arm swinging.

**Perpetuate: Arnold presses:** *4 sets, 15 repetitions.*

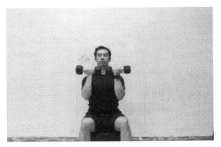
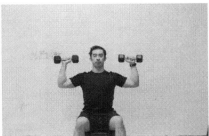
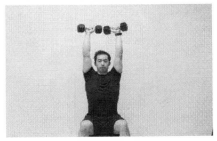

Pro-tip: Move through all 3 phases in a controlled pace and reverse the process on the way down.

# Neck Vertebrae Fracture

**Mobilize: Towel supported neck extensions:** *2 sets, 10 repetitions.*

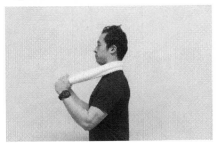
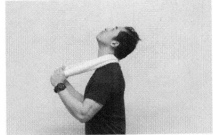

Pro-tip: The towel is there to support the weight of the head and increase the range.

## Mobilize: Towel supported side-flexions: *2 sets, 10 repetitions per side.*

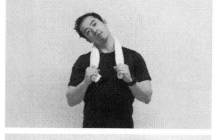

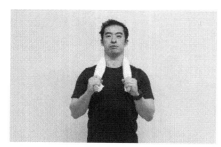

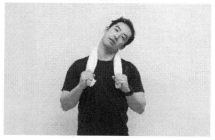

Pro-tip: Try to reach over the towel instead of pressing down into it.

## Mobilize: Towel supported neck rotations: *2 sets, 10 repetitions per side.*

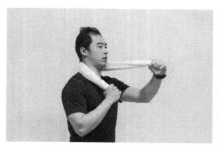

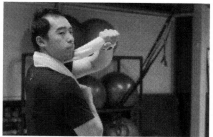

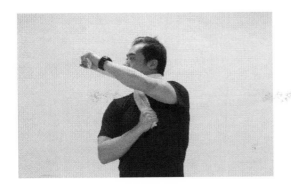

Pro-tip: The top hand is there to assist you to increase the range-of-motion but go as far as pain is tolerated.

## Stabilize: Eccentric focused neck flexion: *2 sets, 10 repetitions.*

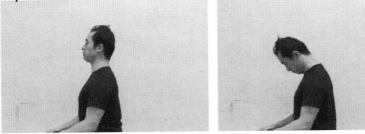

Pro-tip: You are working on the lowering of the head to strengthen the neck and increasing range of motion. Go for 3 seconds down and 3 seconds up.

## Stabilize: Eccentric focused side flexion: *2 sets, 10 repetitions per side.*

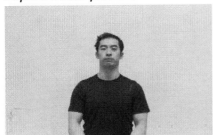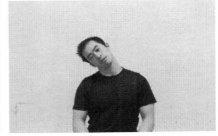

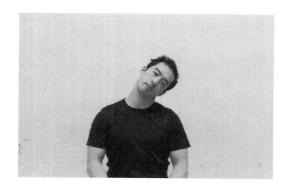

Pro-tip: You are working on the lowering of the head to strengthen the neck and increasing range of motion. Go for 3 seconds down and 3 seconds up.

## Strengthen: Supine neck curl-ups: *3 sets, 10 repetitions.*

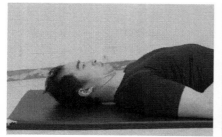 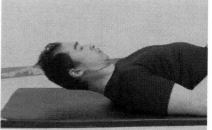

Pro-tip: The stress should be in front of the neck (throat area). There should be very little strain on the back on the neck.

## Strengthen: Quadraped neck extension: *3 sets, 10 repetitions.*

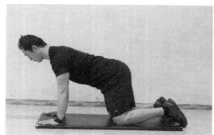 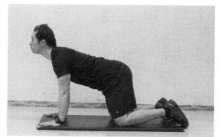

Pro-tip: Keep the shoulders locked downwards as the head comes up.

### Strengthen: Prone Ws: *4 sets, 10 repetitions.*

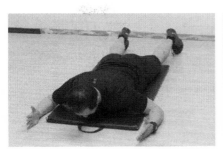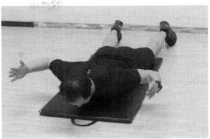

Pro-tip: Lift with the elbows and keep the eyes and head downwards.

### Strengthen: Band Pull-aparts: *4 sets, 15 repetitions.*

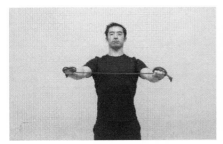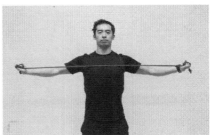

Pro-tip: Keep the shoulders down as you squeeze your shoulder blades together.

### Perpetuate: Bird-dog: *4 sets, 10 repetitions per side.*

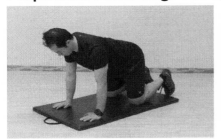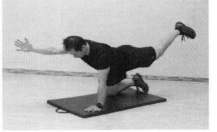

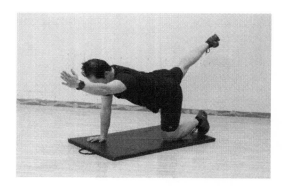

Pro-tip: Keep the eyes downwards as you lift the arm and leg.

**Perpetuate: Waiter's carry:** *4 sets, 45 seconds per arm.*

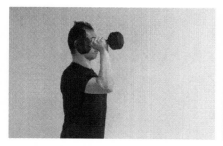 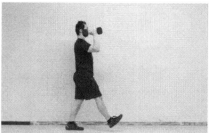

Pro-tip: Keep an upright posture and your shoulder locked as you walk.

**Perpetuate: Wall push-ups:** *4 sets, 10 repetitions.*

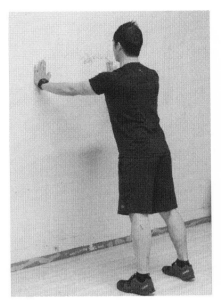 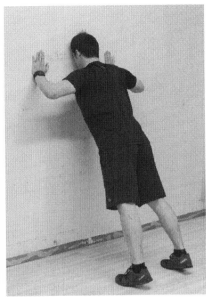

Pro-tip: The elbows should be pointed slightly downwards as you lower into the wall.

# Staple Stretches

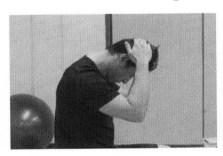 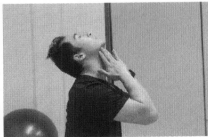

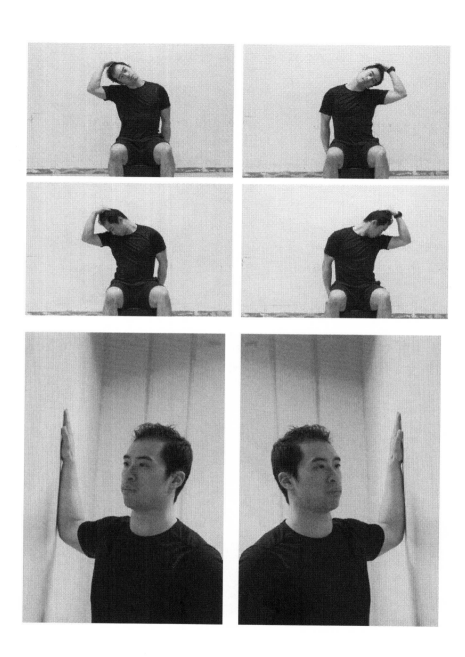

# **5.** Shoulder Injuries

What is a shoulder injury? It could be one or a combination of a bruise, strain, sprain, break or a dislocation that affects a part of your shoulder.

You will most likely feel pain in that area; however, there may be other symptoms which include:

- Lack of mobility in the shoulder with some or all movements.
- Significant weakness in the shoulder compared to the non-injured side.
- "Catching" or cracking sounds when the arm is moved at a certain angle.

The cause of a shoulder injury can come from a magnitude of different sources. Some of which can be:

- Sports such as baseball, golfers, swimmers or athletes who often overuse their arm constantly.
- Acute trauma to the shoulder such as a fall.
- Repetitive actions in the shoulder joint (repetitive strain injury) where you use your shoulder a lot during working hours.
- Muscle imbalances from using one side more than the other.
- Scar tissues developed from a surgery.

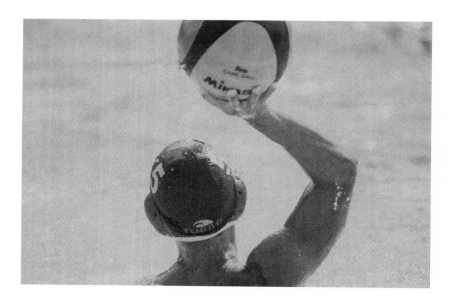

*Chuttersnap (2018).*

Overuse and/or aging can also cause some more complex complications in the shoulder such as:

- **Tendonitis** = inflammation, swelling or micro-tears in a tendon.
- A complete tear is called a **rupture**
- You may get **bursitis,** which is irritation and swelling of a fluid-filled sac that surrounds a joint.
- After so much wear and tear, you may even get **bone spurs** which is extra bone growth in the joint.

So who is most likely to suffer? Because the shoulder is used in almost everything we do, individuals with labour-heavy jobs are affected. Some occupations include computer operators, construction workers, dentists, painters, hair-dressers, etc. These jobs have a high rate of repetitive strain injury because their shoulder is active almost all of the time they are working.

**Shoulder Science**

The shoulder joint is essentially a ball-and-socket joint that connects the upper arm to the trunk; also known as the glenohumeral joint. It is commonly known that this joint is one of the more "fragile" joint because it can move in all directions, like a Swiffer. Because of the increased flexibility of this joint, there is also an increased chance of injury (if no pre-hab is performed regularly).

Three bone structures are located in this region:

- The humerus: the bone in the upper arm.
- The scapula: the shoulder blade.
- The clavicle: the collarbone.

A few soft-tissue components also make up the shoulder joint:

- Rotator cuff muscles and ligaments (VERY IMPORTANT).
- Tendons to connect muscle-to-bone; ligaments that connect bone-to-bone.
- Bursa, a fluid-filled sac that acts like a lubricant to prevent any rubbing inside the shoulder joint.
- A fascia which is a huge band that attaches and encloses all these structures together.

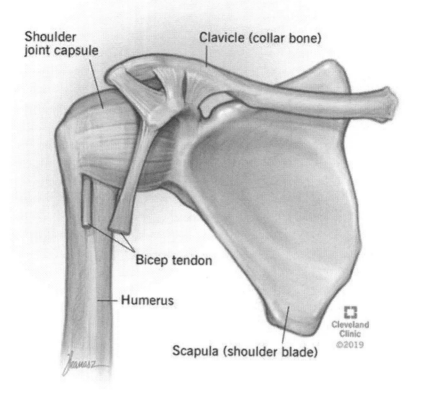

*Thompson (2019).*

## Rotator Cuff Muscles

These muscles are a group of four distinct muscles and their tendon, responsible for specific shoulder movements. These include: supraspinatus, infraspinatus, teres minor and subscapularis. These muscles begin at the scapula (shoulder blade) and connect to the humerus forming a "cuff" around the joint.

With active rehab treatment, we significantly target these muscles in order to re-create the stability it once had.

Different movements at the shoulder joint can target specific muscles in the rotator cuff. It is crucial that we are able to diagnose which muscles has been compromise in order to prescribe the appropriate exercise.

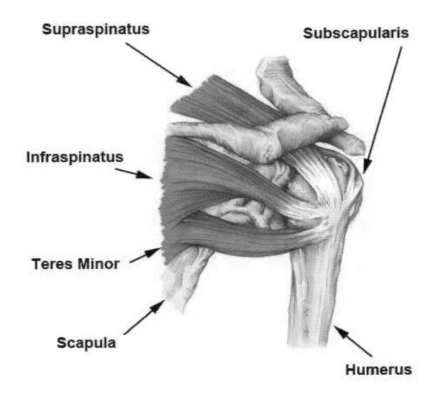

*Williams (2019).*

<u>Rotator Cuff TEAR?</u>

This injury is often tricky because it is quite difficult to pinpoint the actual location of the rotator cuff tear. You may need the guidance of a physiotherapist for this one. Generally this injury occurs with sudden trauma or repetitive actions. With older individuals, movements such as reaching overhead may cause pain in the shoulder as well. Most rotator cuff tears do not require surgery but they can take an extended amount of time to recover as the supporting structures are complex in nature.

To treat it, we follow the system. First stabilize and mobilize, then strengthen. Because most of the time we are not sure of the exact muscle that is torn, we would target the shoulder at every angle in order to cover as much area as we can. During exercise therapy, if there is any "shooting" pain, you must slow down or stop because this could cause further damage.

SLAP who? SLAP tear.

This is short for "superior labrum anterior or posterior" tear. The labrum is the ring that runs around the cavity of the scapula connecting the head of the humerus. A SLAP tear, is when this surrounding tissue rips. The tear can occur on top, in front or behind the socket. The SLAP tear is common in athletes who have repetitive overhead motion, such as baseball and tennis players.

I would recommend focus more attention on the stability part of the system rather than the mobility part. Of course, both are important; however, we must consider the function of the labrum in the shoulder – stabilization. In order to restore its function, we must boost it by focusing on stability movements.

## What is the difference between shoulder dislocation and separation?

The difference between the two injuries begins at the location where the injury happened. A shoulder separation happens when there is an injury to the ligament between the shoulder blade and collarbone. This may even cause a bump in the affected area. Some symptoms may include pain, swelling, bruising and limited motion.

# Separated Shoulder

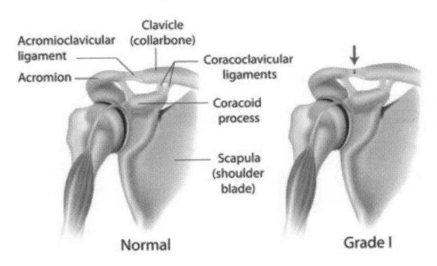

*The shoulder clinic of Idaho (2020).*

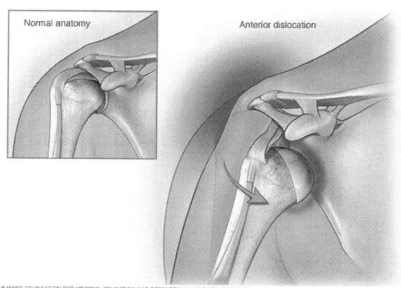

Normal anatomy

Anterior dislocation

*Mayo Clinic Staff (2020).*

A shoulder dislocation, however, occurs when the top of the arm bone loses contact with the socket of the shoulder blade and comes apart. Symptoms can include severe shoulder pain, arm positioned away from the body and deformity just below the shoulder.

### Got the chills? Frozen shoulder?

Technical name: adhesive capsulitis. This is something that will impact all aspects of your life as it gets very restrictive in your ball-and-socket joint. You may experience pain, progressive stiffness and/or decrease in range-of-motion. This immobilization usually happens after extended time of little movement, an injury or experiencing conditions such as diabetes, hyperthyroidism and Parkinson's.

Within the ball-and-socket joint is a liquid called the synovial fluid. The job of this fluid is to keep the joint lubricated and allows for smooth, gliding movements. With frozen shoulder, the synovial fluid thickens and becomes inflamed, which ultimately causes the joint to become extremely rigid. The inflammation leaves less space for the humerus to move – giving it a "frozen" or "limited" feeling.

One notable point: the capsule by itself is not very strong. However, it is guarded by several rotator cuff muscles that provide the stability needed for every day functions.

# Treatments

## Frozen Shoulder

**Mobilize: Dowel flexion & scapular depression:** *2 sets, 10 repetitions.*

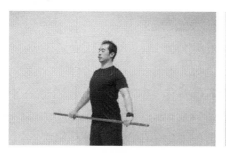 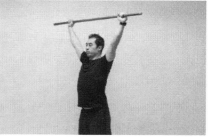

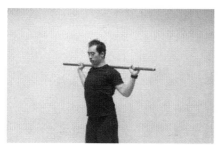

Pro-tip: Go to the maximum range at the highest point before bringing the dowel down.

## Mobilize: Towel glides: *2 sets, 10 repetitions for bottom and top.*

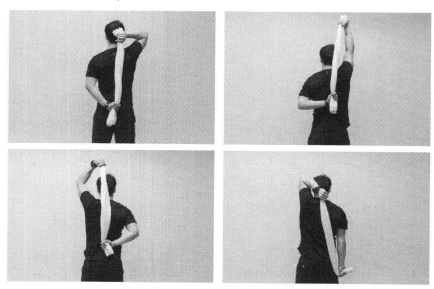

Pro-tip: Pictures shown is a left arm focused. Above picture works on internal rotation while the bottom picture works on external rotation.

## Mobilize: Dynamic sleeper stretch: *2 sets, 5 repetitions.*

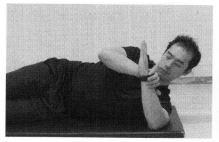 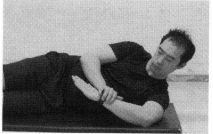

Pro-tip: Make it a fluid and smooth motion; aim for 3 seconds down and 3 seconds up.

**Stabilize: Plank plus:** *3 sets, 10 repetitions.*

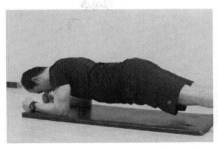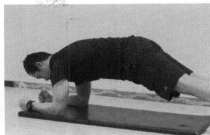

Pro-tip: The movement is at the shoulder blades; squeezing on the way down and opening on the way up.

**Stabilize: Prone single press-ups:** *3 sets, 10 repetitions.*

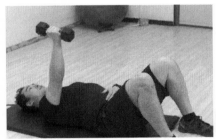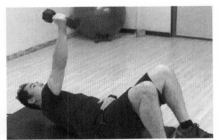

Pro-tip: This is a small movement by lifting the shoulder off the floor.

**Stabilize: Ball wall circles:** *3 sets, 10 repetition per direction.*

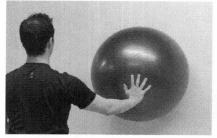 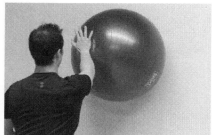

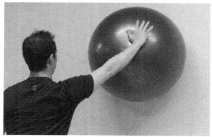

Pro-tip: Keep shoulder locked back and down into place while the circles are being made.

**Strengthen: Band external & internal rotations:** *4 sets, 15 repetitions each.*

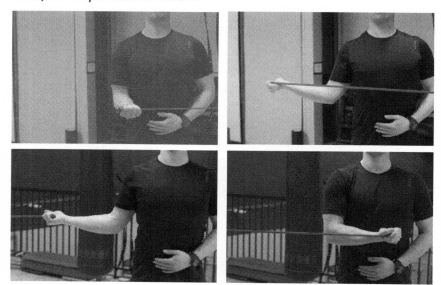

Pro-tip: The top two pictures the hand is moving away from the body and toward the body for the bottom two pictures. Keep the shoulder back and locked downwards as you move through the movement.

## **Strengthen: Finger walk to shoulder flexion:** *4 sets, 10 repetitions.*

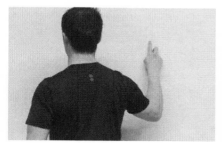
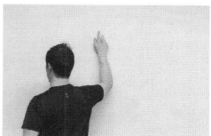
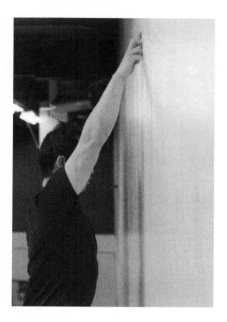

Pro-tip: The walking of the fingers is aimed to give you some assistance with shoulder flexion.

### Strengthen: Prone A: *4 sets, 15 repetitions.*

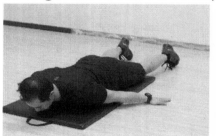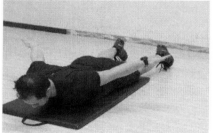

Pro-tip: Squeeze the shoulder blades and lift by the elbows.

### Perpetuate: Dumbbell rows: *4 sets, 15 repetitions.*

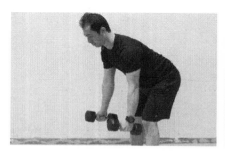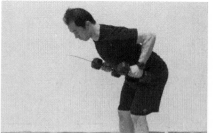

Pro-tip: Keep the elbows close to the body and keep the back straight and good posture.

### Perpetuate: Band lateral raises: *4 sets, 15 repetitions per side.*

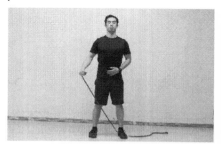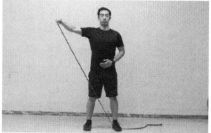

Pro-tip: Keep the shoulder locked in place while you raise the band.

**Perpetuate: Dumbbell shoulder press:** *4 sets, 15 repetitions.*

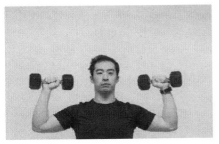 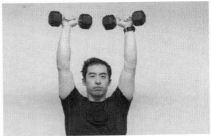

Pro-tip: Keep good posture at the top of the movement.

## Shoulder Labral Tear

**Mobilize: Dowel Kayak extensions:** *2 sets, 10 repetitions per side.*

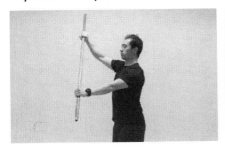 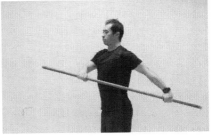

Pro-tip: Drive the arm back as far as pain is tolerated, working on extension.

## Mobilize: **Corkscrew:** *2 sets, 5 repetition per side.*

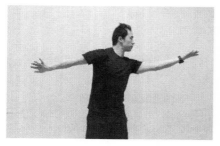 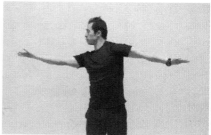

Pro-tip: Twist the arm is far as pain is tolerated and keep the motions fluid and controlled.

## Mobilize: **Arm reaches: 2 sets, 5 repetitions per arm.**

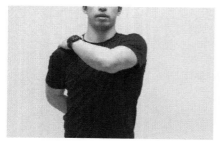 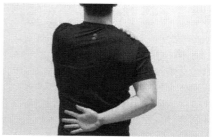

Pro-tip: Reach as far as pain is tolerated.

## Stabilize: **High plank:** *3 sets, 45 seconds - 1 minute hold.*

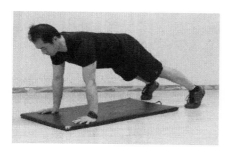

Pro-tip: Keep the shoulders locked back and down, and stacked over the elbow.

## Stabilize: Waiter's carry: *3 sets, 45 seconds of walk.*

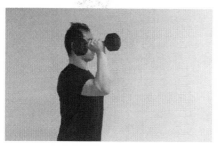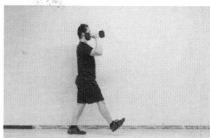

Pro-tip: Lift the weight by the elbow and keep the shoulders locked downward.

## Stabilize: Isometric external rotation with walk-out: *3 sets, 10 steps per arm.*

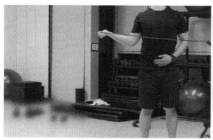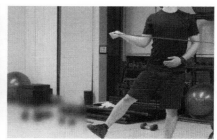

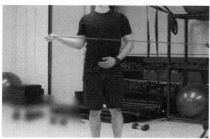

Pro-tip: It is one step out and one step in for one repetition and keep the elbow locked at 90 degrees and tight to the body.

## Strengthen: Band flexion & abduction: *4 sets: 10 repetitions each.*

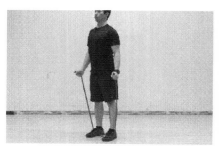
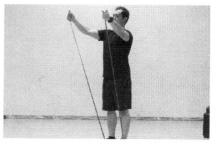
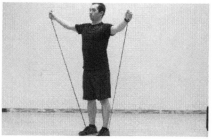

Pro-tip: Stand tall with shoulders back and down as you raise the band.

## Strengthen: Prone Y, T, W, A: *4 sets, 10 of each letter.*

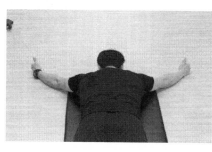
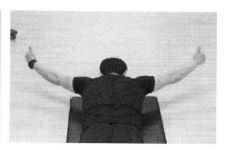
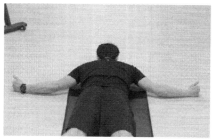
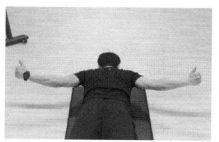

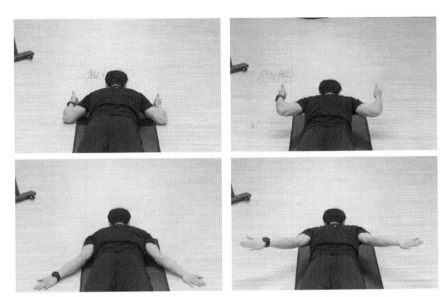

Pro-tip: Shoulder blades are squeezed with shoulders down with all shapes.

## Strengthen: Sword draw: *4 sets, 15 repetitions per arm.*

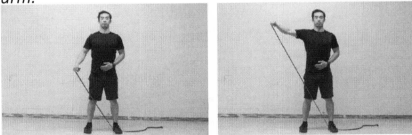

Pro-tip: Lift the band by the elbows.

**Perpetuate: Shoulder focused push-ups:** *4 sets, 10 repetitions.*

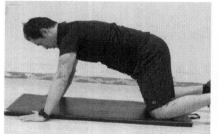 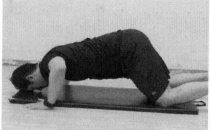

Pro-tip: Rock the hips back to target more of the shoulders.

**Perpetuate: Underarm pull-downs:** *4 sets, 15 repetitions.*

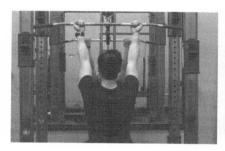 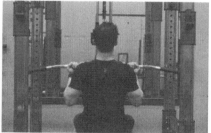

Pro-tip: Keep the shoulders down throughout the entire movement.

**Perpetuate: Bar shoulder press:** *4 sets, 15 repetitions*

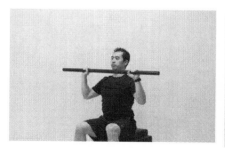 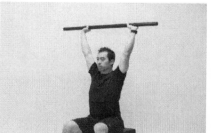

Pro-tips: Drive the bar up until it ends up directly above the head.

# Shoulder Bursitis

**Mobilize: Scapular rolls:** *2 sets, 10 repetitions forward then backward.*

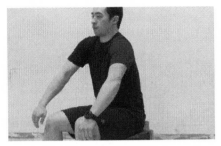 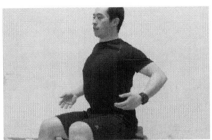

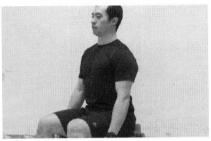

Pro-tip: Get the arms involved to get a bigger range-of-motion. Go slowly.

**Mobilize: Dynamic reach-over-shoulder:** *2 sets, 5 repetitions per side.*

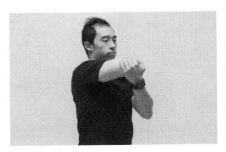 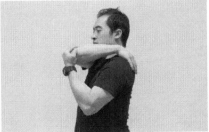

Pro-tip: Keep the movements smooth and controlled.

## Mobilize: Dumbbell pendulum circles: *2 sets, 10 rotations per side per arm.*

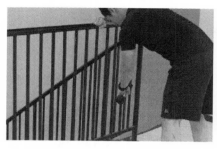 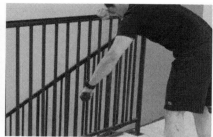

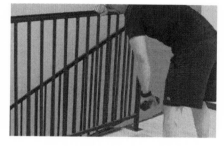

Pro-tip: Drop the shoulder a bit and completely relax the arm.

**Stabilize: Isometric external rotation:** *3 sets, 45 seconds per arm.*

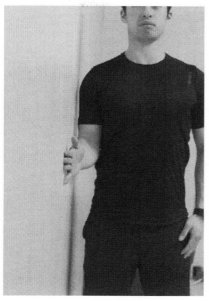

Pro-tip: Push outwards as hard as you can for the duration of the set, keeping the elbows locked at 90 degrees.

**Stabilize: Isometric internal rotation,** *3 sets, 45 seconds per arm.*

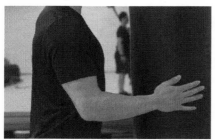

Pro-tip: Push inwards as hard as you can for the duration of the set, keeping the elbows locked at 90 degrees.

**Stabilize: Side plank,** *2 sets 45 seconds each side.*

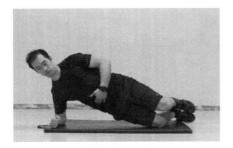

Pro-tip: Keep the shoulder locked down and keep the head away from the shoulders.

**Strengthen: Prone single press-ups:** *4 sets, 10 repetition per side.*

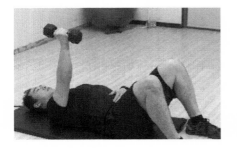 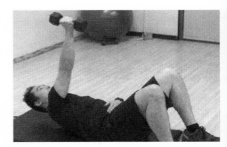

Pro-tip: It is a small movement. Lift until the shoulder comes off the floor then stop.

**Strengthen: Standing dowel flexion + extension:** *4 sets, 10 repetitions for flexion and 10 repetitions for extension per set.*

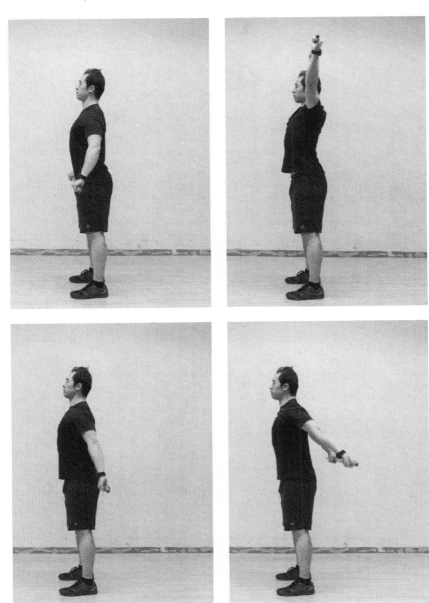

Pro-tip: Do 10 forward with straight arm, then behind your back for 10.

### Strengthen: Dowel press-outs: *4 sets, 15 repetitions.*

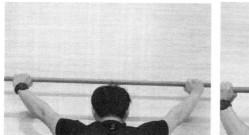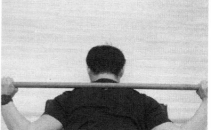

Pro-tip: Try to get the elbows locked out without putting the hands on the ground.

### Perpetuate: Single dumbbell rows: *4 sets, 15 repetitions.*

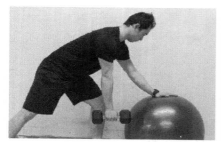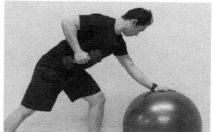

Pro-tip: It is fine to go heavier for this movement as long as your keeping the shoulder locked in.

**Perpetuate: Dumbbell lateral raises:** *4 sets, 15 repetitions.*

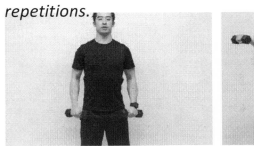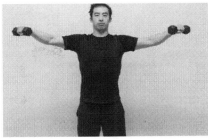

Pro-tip: You may need to go slightly lighter because it is specifically targeting the shoulders.

**Perpetuate: Inch-worms:** *4 sets, 10 repetitions.*

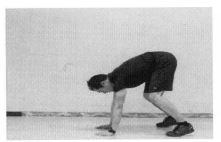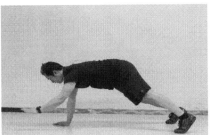

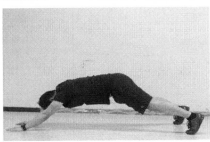

Pro-tip: The farther you go with your hands, the more stress will be put on the shoulders so go as far as pain will allow it.

# Shoulder (AC) Separation

**Mobilize: Standing dowel external rotation:** *2 sets, 10 repetitions per side.*

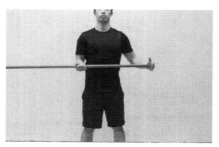 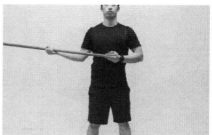

Pro-tip: In the image the right arm is the focused side so the left arm is responsible for assisting the towel into external rotation.

**Mobilize: Screw drivers:** *2 sets, 10 repetitions per side.*

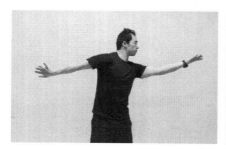 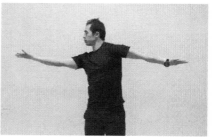

Pro-tip: Turn the palms as high or back as you can.

**Mobilize: Open book:** *2 sets, 10 repetitions per side.*

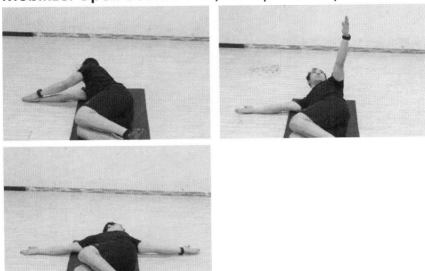

Pro-tip: Keep the knees and hips from moving, and eyes on the moving hand.

**Stabilize: 3-point shoe holds:** *2 sets, each point is held for 30 seconds.*

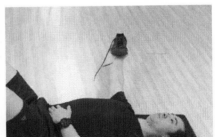

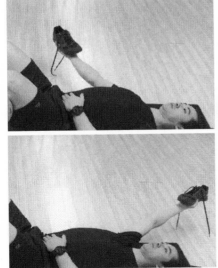

Pro-tip: Each set consists of 5 low, 5 middle and 5 high point. Keep the shoulder locked into place.

## Stabilize: Shoulder taps: *2 sets, 10 repetitions per side.*

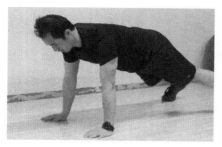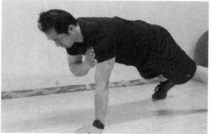

Pro-tip: Keep the shoulder stacked on top of the elbow and wrist, and keep it stiff.

## Stabilize: Band wall walk-ups: *2 sets, 10 repetitions.*

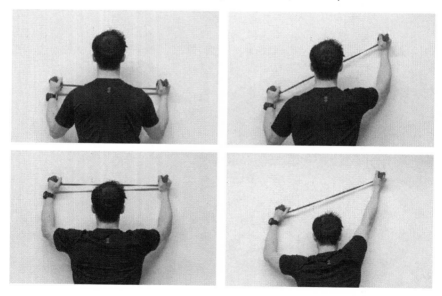

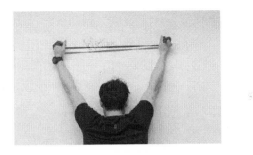

Pro-tip: Each full completion of an up and down is one repetition. Keep the shoulders back and down throughout the entire movement.

## Strengthen: Plank plus: *4 sets, 10 repetitions.*

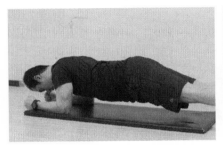 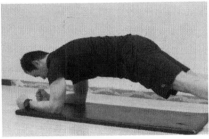

Pro-tip: The movement is at the shoulder blades; it folds in and out during the movement.

**Strengthen: Sword draw:** *4 sets, 15 repetitions per arm.*

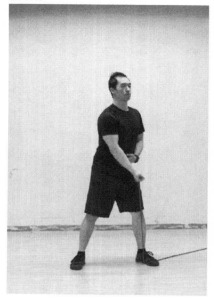 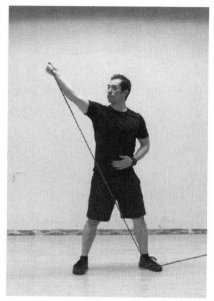

Pro-tip: Make sure the arm crosses the body and ends up next to your head.

**Strengthen: Band Y+T+A:** *4 sets, 10 repetitions per letter.*

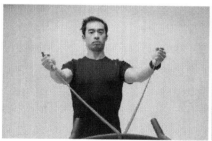 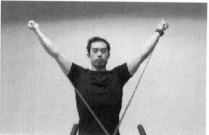

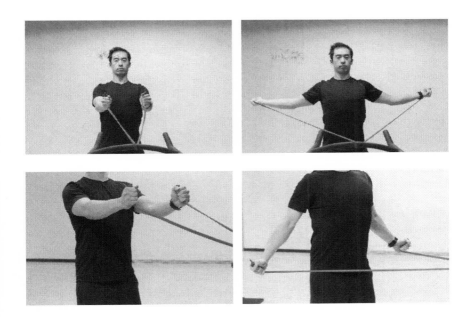

Pro-tip: Shoulders are peeled back at all times; the focus is on the upper back.

**Perpetuate: Dumbbell rows:** *4 sets, 15 repetitions.*

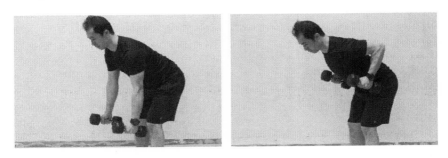

Pro-tip: You may row heavier as long as you can keep your back straight and posture in-check.

**Perpetuate: Bear crawls:** *4 sets, 45 seconds of crawl.*

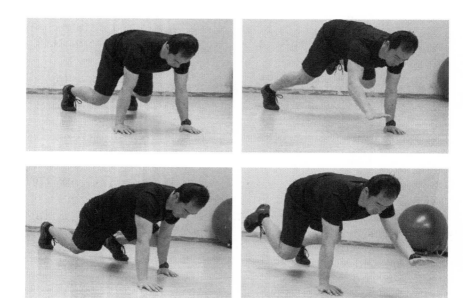

Pro-tip: Keep your hips down as you crawl. The movement is slow and controlled; focusing on the shoulders.

**Perpetuate: Push-ups:** *4 sets, 10 repetitions.*

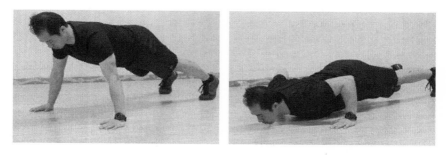

Pro-tip: You may start on your knees then progress onto your toes.

# Shoulder dislocation

**Mobilize: Dumbbell pendulum swing:** *2 sets, 10 repetitions per direction per arm.*

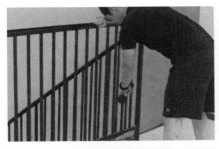
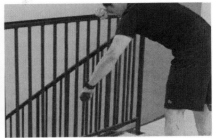
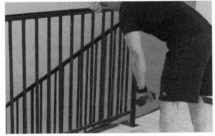

Pro-tip: Drop the shoulder a bit and completely relax the arm.

**Mobilize: Dynamic sleeper stretch:** *2 sets, 10 repetitions per arm.*

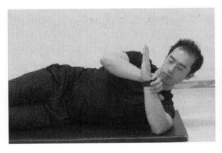
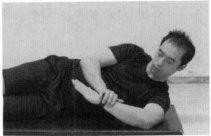

Pro-tip: Keep the movement fluid and controlled.

**Mobilize: Pectoral stretch slides:** *2 sets, 10 repetitions per arm.*

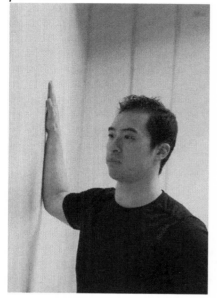 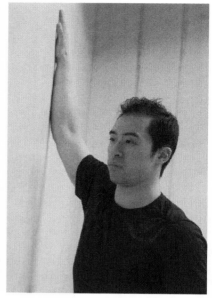

Pro-tip: Slide the arm up slowly. You should also feel a stretch in the chest area.

**Stabilize: Static ball press:** *3 sets, 45 seconds of hold.*

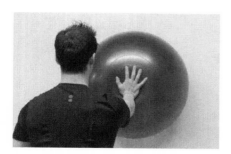

Pro-tip: Press into the ball as hard as you can keeping the shoulder locked back and down.

**Stabilize: Shoulder extension:** *3 sets, 10 repetitions.*

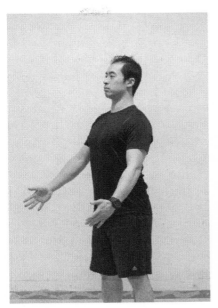 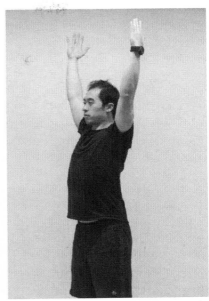

Pro-tip: Make sure you lift both arms to the same height without arching your back.

**Stabilize: Isometric scapulae squeeze:** *3 sets, 45 seconds of hold.*

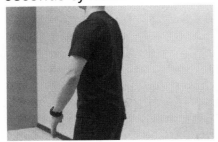 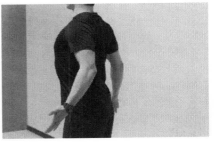

Pro-tip: The hold is at the shoulder blades and turn the palms forward.

## Strengthen: Finger walk to shoulder flexion: 4 sets, 10 repetitions.

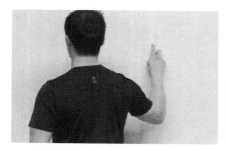 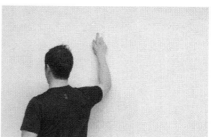

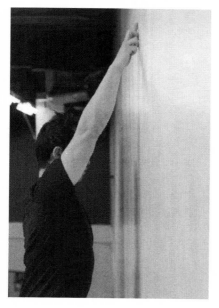

Pro-tip: The point of the "walking fingers" is to assist the arm into flexion.

**Strengthen: Band external & internal rotation:** *4 sets, 15 repetitions of each.*

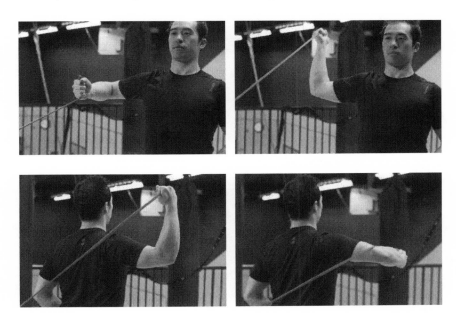

Pro-tip: The above picture is external rotation; below is internal rotation.

**Strengthen: Bent-over wing-spans:** *4 sets, 15 repetitions.*

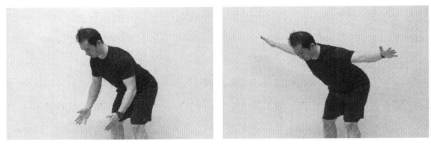

Pro-tip: Keep the shoulder blades together at all times and move the arm in a controlled manner.

**Strengthen: Wall wipe crosses:** *4 sets, 10 repetitions.*

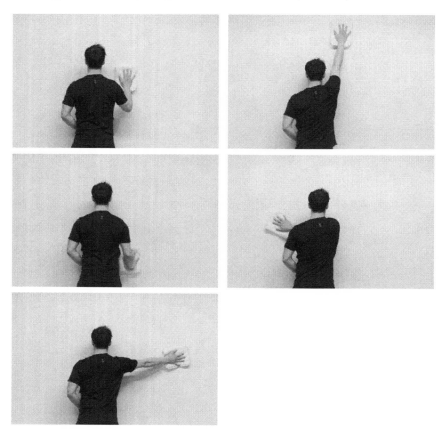

Pro-tip: Each time a cross is made is one repetition. Be sure to extend to the end range in each direction.

**Perpetuate: Cable face-pulls:** *4 sets, 15 repetitions.*

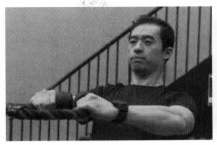 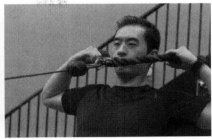

Pro-tip: Keep shoulders back and pull by the elbows.

**Perpetuate: Overhead carries:** *4 sets, 45 seconds of walk.*

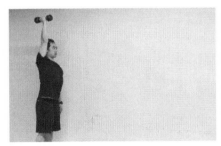 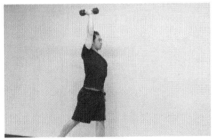

Pro-tip: Don't let the shoulder come loose during the walk.

**Perpetuate: Push-ups:** *4 sets, 15 repetitions.*

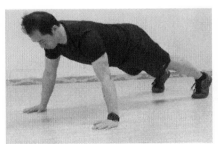 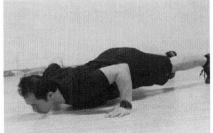

Pro-tip: You may begin on your knees then process onto the toes.

# Shoulder Blade Pain

**Mobilize: Quadraped rotation with reach:** *2 sets, 10 repetitions per side.*

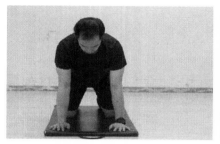 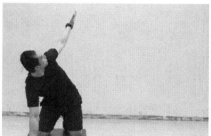

Pro-tip: Rotate the body as you reach with the arm.

**Mobilize: Quadraped with overhead reach:** *2 sets, 10 repetitions per arm.*

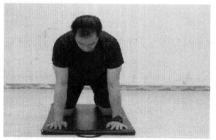 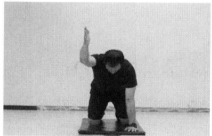

Pro-tip: Keep the head and body still; lift the arm at the shoulders.

## Mobilize: **Prone reach-downs:** *2 sets, 10 repetitions.*

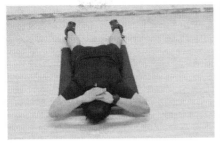 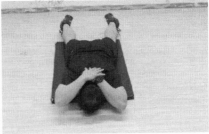

Pro-tip: Reach down the spine with two hands then return to the back of the head.

## Stabilize: **Side planks:** *3 sets, 10 repetitions per side.*

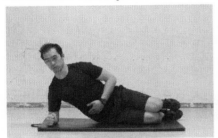 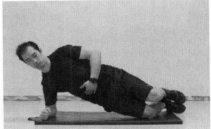

Pro-tip: Keep the shoulder and trunk stiff as you lift the hips off the ground.

## Stabilize: **Shoulder taps:** *3 sets, 5 repetitions per arm.*

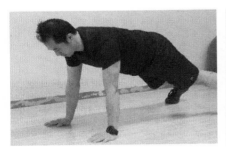 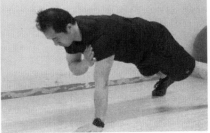

Pro-tip: Keep the shoulder stiff and locked down throughout the set.

### Stabilize: Scapulae push-ups: *3 sets, 10 repetitions.*

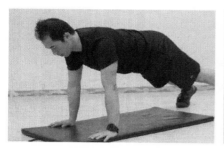 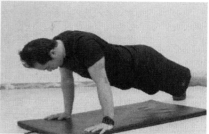

Pro-tip: The movement is at the shoulder blades, folding in and out.

### Strengthen: Wall arm slides - parallel + Y: *4 sets, 10 repetitions each.*

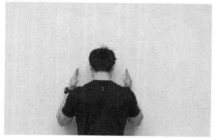 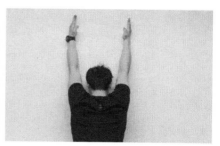

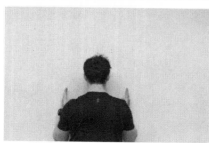 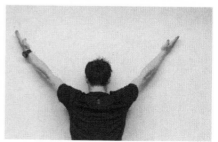

Pro-tip: Do 10 of the first shape, then 10 of the Y - that is one set. Move fluidly.

**Strengthen: Prone W:** *4 sets, 15 repetitions.*

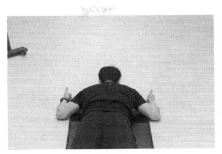 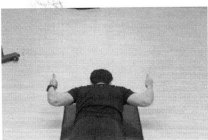

Pro-tip: Keep the shoulder blades back and down as you lift the elbows up.

**Strengthen: Band external rotations:** *4 sets, 15 repetitions.*

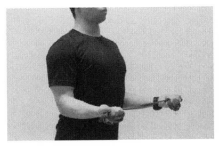 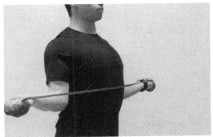

Pro-tip: Keep the shoulder blades back and rotate the arms outward.

**Strengthen: Band overhead reaches:** *4 sets, 15 repetitions.*

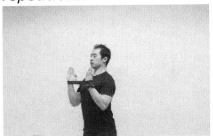 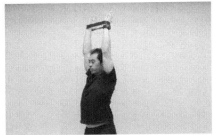

Pro-tip: Keep the band under tension as you reach above head.

### Perpetuate: Bent-over reverse flies: *4 sets, 15 repetitions.*

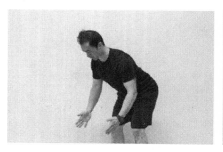 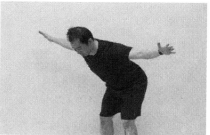

Pro-tip: Keep the back straight and the shoulders back. Add weight for progression.

### Perpetuate: Renegade rows: *4 sets, 5 repetitions per arm.*

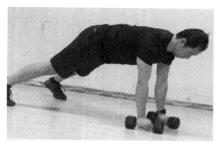 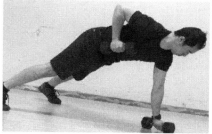

Pro-tip: Keep the shoulders and trunk stiff throughout the movement.

**Perpetuate: Dumbbell shoulder press:** *4 sets, 15 repetitions.*

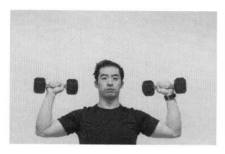 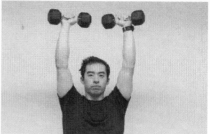

Pro-tip: You can choose a heavier weight for this movement when strength is built up.

# Biceps Tendon Tear

**Mobilize: Dynamic sleeper stretch:** *2 sets, 10 repetitions per side.*

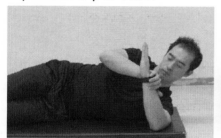 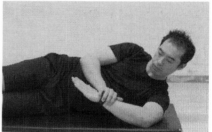

Pro-tip: Keep the entire movement fluid and controlled.

**Mobilize: Bicep wall stretch:** *2 sets, 45 seconds per side.*

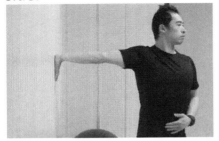

Pro-tip: Open up the chest and shoulder for an increased stretch.

**Mobilize: Wrist extensor stretch:** *2 sets, 10 repetitions per side.*

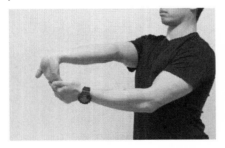

Pro-tip: Keep the elbow locked for the best stretch.

**Stabilize: High planks:** *3 sets, 45 seconds per set.*

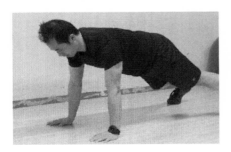

Pro-tip: Keep the shoulder stacked over the elbow and wrist, forming a straight line.

### Stabilize: Triceps push-down: *3 sets, 20 repetitions.*

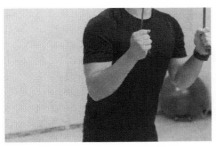 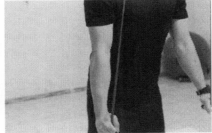

Pro-tip: Lock out your arms at the bottom of the movement.

### Stabilize: Dumbbell supinate/pronate: 3 sets, 15 repetitions.

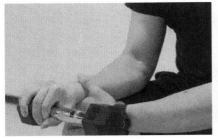 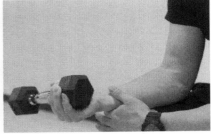

Pro-tip: Keep the wrist flat and turn the dumbbell as far as pain allows it.

## Strengthen: Band external/internal rotation: *3 sets, 20 repetitions per direction.*

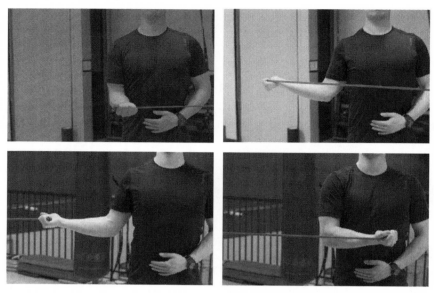

Pro-tip: The above picture shows moving the arm outward while the bottom shows pulling the band inward.

## Strengthen: Bent-over band shoulder extension: 3 sets, 20 repetitions.

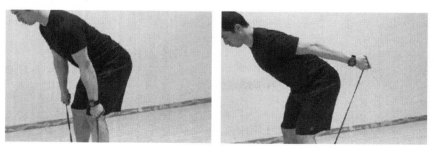

Pro-tip: Lift by the elbows and keep the shoulder locked downwards.

### Strengthen: Dumbbell front raises: *3 sets, 15 repetitions.*

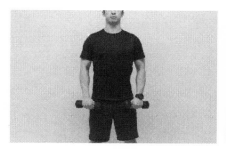 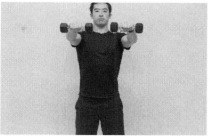

Pro-tip: Keep the entire movement under controlled with no swinging.

### Strengthen: Dumbbell bicep curls + reverse curls: *3 sets, 20 repetitions.*

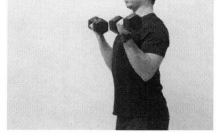

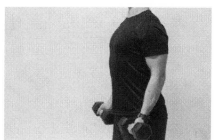

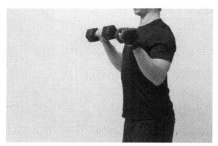

Pro-tip: Choose a weight that you can do the entire set without stopping.

**Perpetuate: Barbell bench press:** *4 sets, 10 repetitions.*

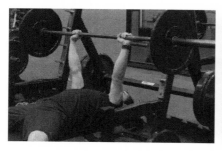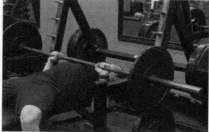

Pro-tip: Choose a weight that allows you to get full range-of-motion.

**Perpetuate: Barbell bent-over rows:** *4 sets, 10 repetitions.*

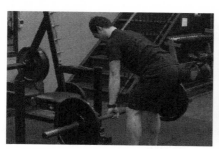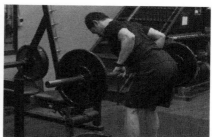

Pro-tip: You can go heavier to really stress the elbow.

**Perpetuate: Band hammer curls: 4 sets, 20 repetitions.**

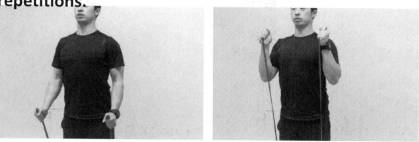

Pro-tip: You are going for muscular endurance here so it will burn.

## Staple Stretches

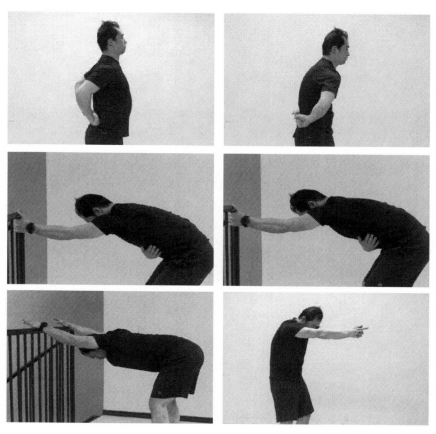

# 6. Elbow, wrist & hand injuries

## Elbow issues

In my experience treating elbow pain, the cause of it is either bracing a fall or from overuse. Of course there can be many other reasons but trauma or repetitive strain is popular. More severe cases can include fractures of different anatomical structures.

Various symptoms of an elbow fracture include pain, swelling, bruising and/or stiffness. At the time of the injury, an audible sound, such as a pop or snap, might be heard. If the elbow looks "deformed", it may mean that the bones are out of place and possibly dislocated. And almost all the time, the elbow and arm will feel numb or weak.

Severe fractures that are out of place and unstable, should be consulted with a surgeon or specialist. Bone fragments that result from the fracture need to be surgically removed, otherwise they create further complications. Less severe fractures may use non-surgical treatment, like a cast or split, to keep it in place for recovery.

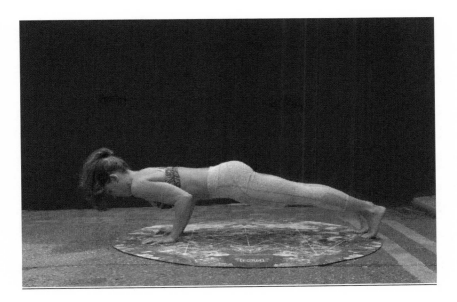

*Form (2017).*

## Tennis vs. Golfer's Elbow

This does not only come from playing tennis or golf, other activities can lead to it too. Both injuries usually result from the repetitive strain on the tendons.

Tennis elbow is often characterized as pain coming from the outside of the elbow (on the lateral epicondyle). This pain may travel down to the forearm and back of the hand when grasping or twisting.

Golfer's elbow is pain coming from the inside of the elbow (affecting tendons connecting to the medial epicondyle).

Common symptoms from both injuries include:

- Pain or tenderness in the elbow region.
- Weakness in the forearm, wrist, hand or grip.

119

- Pain when you grip an object, twist things and/or wave an object around.
- Could be some shooting pain down the forearm into the hands and fingers.

Usually these injuries start gradually and get worse as time goes on.

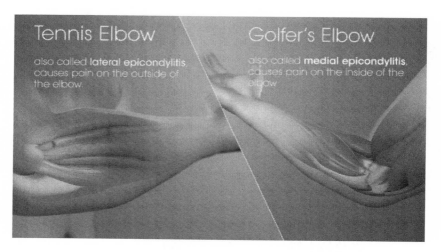

*Khera (2016).*

## Carpal Tunnel Syndrome

This is a common condition that causes pain, numbness and tingling in the hands and arm. You may feel occasional "shock-like" sensation that shoots down into the hand. You may even feel like dropping things due to weakness in the wrist and hand. This is caused by one of the major nerve (that runs into the hand) being compressed. Similar to tennis and golfer's elbow, carpal tunnel syndrome gets worse over time.

Which nerve gets compressed? It is the median nerve. If the pressure continues it can lead to nerve damage. To prevent permanent damage, surgery may be recommended. Carpal tunnel syndrome occurs when the "tunnel" becomes narrowed or when the surrounding tissues (called the synovium) swell up and squeezes the median nerve. The synovium lubricates the tendons ensuring smooth finger movements. However, swelling of the synovium will cause pain, numbness or weakness in the hand.

Some causes can be:

- Heredity: genes can be passed on and can run in families.
- Repetitive hand use: using your hand a lot in the same way is a good way to develop carpal tunnel syndrome.
- Hand and wrist position: having the wrist in extreme flexion and extension for a prolonged period of time can increase pressure on the median nerve.
- Health conditions: Diabetes, thyroid and arthritis are associated with carpal tunnel syndrome.

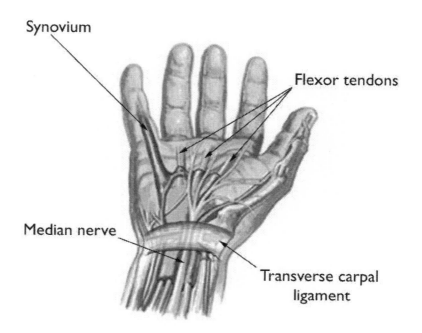

Synovium

Flexor tendons

Median nerve

Transverse carpal ligament

*Orthoinfo (2020).*

<u>Wrist, hand and finger rehabilitation</u>

We must be extra cautious during rehabilitation with the hand region because structures are particularly fragile. Majority of the rehab revolves around increasing grip strength and wrist stability when loaded. Of course our system must be followed in order to ensure maximum recovery. Because we use our wrist, hand and fingers in our everyday lives, it becomes a double-edged sword.

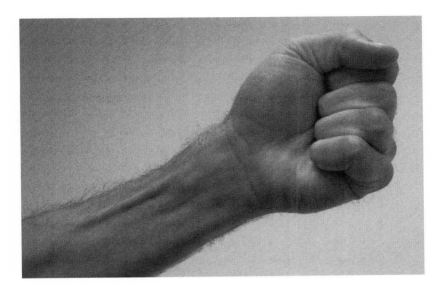

*Noble (2019).*

## Treatments

## Golfer's Elbow

**Mobilize: Lacrosse ball smash on elbow (inside + outside):** *2 sets, 45 seconds.*

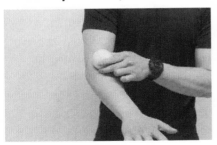 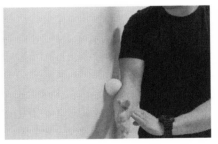

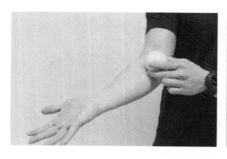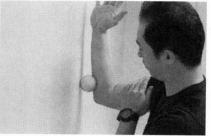

Pro-tip: Avoid any bony areas and massage until the area has loosened up.

## Stabilize: Elbow plank: *3 sets, 45 seconds per set.*

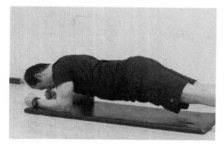

Pro-tip: If there is too much stress on the elbow, you can put your knees down.

## Stabilize: High plank: *3 sets, 45 seconds per set.*

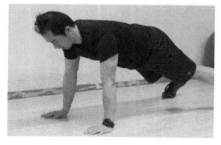

Pro-tip: You can begin on the knees then progress on the toes for progression.

### Stabilize: Grip strengthening: Dumbbell gripping: *3 sets, 45 seconds of hold.*

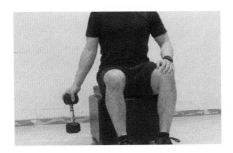

Pro-tip: Pick a weight that you can sustain the entire 45 seconds.

### Strengthen: Triceps push-downs: *4 sets, 20 repetitions.*

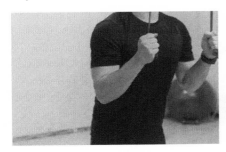 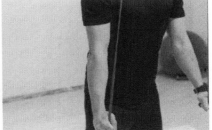

Pro-tip: Lock out the arms at the bottom of the movement.

**Strengthen: Dumbbell supination + pronation:** *4 sets, 10 repetitions.*

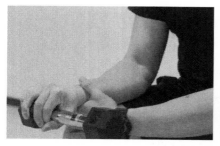 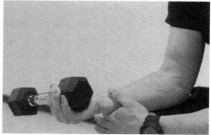

Pro-tip: Keep the wrists flat and move through full range-of-motion.

**Strengthen: Band curls: supinated, hammer + pronated:** *3 set, 20 repetition of each grip.*

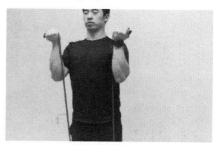

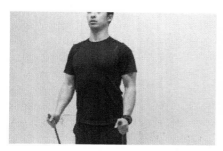 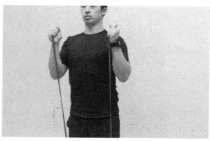

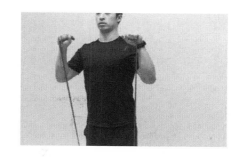

Pro-tip: Do 20 repetition of the bicep curl, then 20 repetition of the hammer curl, then 20 repetition of the reverse curl. That is one set.

## Strengthen: Face-pulls: *4 sets, 15 repetitions.*

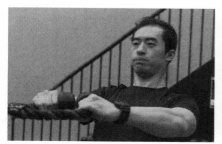 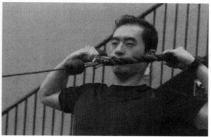

Pro-tip: Pull by the elbows and squeeze the shoulder blades together.

## Perpetuate: Floor press: *4 sets, 15 repetitions.*

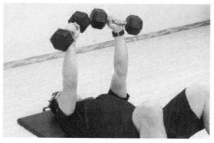 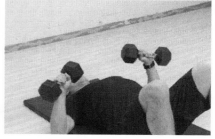

Pro-tip: Control the weight on the way down and ensure the elbows touch the floor.

## Perpetuate: Dumbbell curls: *4 sets, 15 repetitions.*

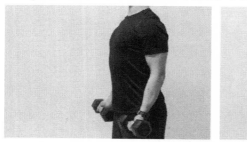 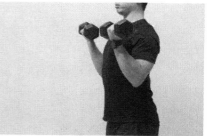

Pro-tip: You may pick a heavier weight to further stress the elbow.

## Perpetuate: Dumbbell rows: *4 sets, 15 repetitions.*

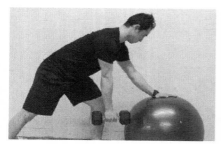 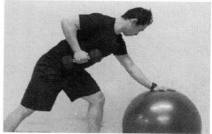

Pro-tip: You may choose a heavier weight to further stress the elbow joint.

# Tennis Elbow

**Mobilize: Dynamic tricep stretch:** *2 sets, 10 repetitions per side.*

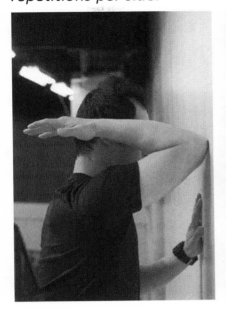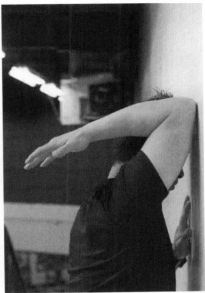

Pro-tip: Slide as high as pain will allow it and keep the movement controlled and fluid.

**Mobilize: Lacrosse ball smash on outer elbow:** *2 sets, 45 seconds per side.*

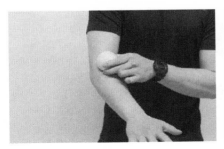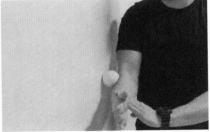

Pro-tip: Avoid any bony structures and massage until the area has loosened up.

### Stabilize: Grip strengthening: *3 sets, 45 seconds each hand.*

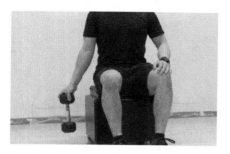

Pro-tip: Choose a weight that you can hold for the entire 45 seconds.

### Stabilize: Towel carries: *3 sets, 45 seconds of walk per hand.*

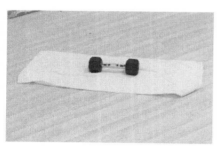 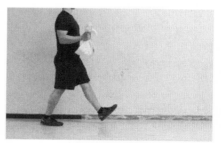

Pro-tip: Keep the elbow locked at 90 degrees and avoid any swinging.

**Strengthen: Wrist flexion and extension:** *4 sets, 10 repetitions of each.*

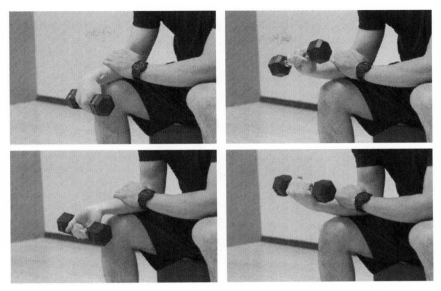

Pro-tip: Do 10 of palms-down, then 10 of palms-up; that is 1 set. Keep all movements slow and controlled.

**Strengthen: Wrist supinate & pronate:** *4 sets, 10 repetitions.*

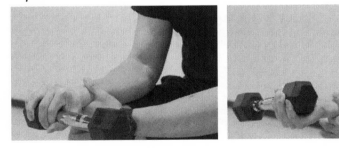

Pro-tip: Keep all movements fluid and controlled. Try to get as much range as possible.

**Strengthen: Band upright rows:** *4 sets, 15 repetitions.*

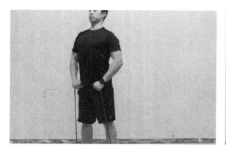 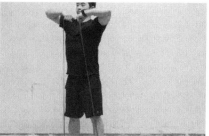

Pro-tip: Keep the shoulders peeled back and pull by the elbows.

**Strengthen: Dumbbell skull-crushers:** *4 sets, 15 repetitions.*

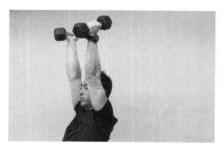 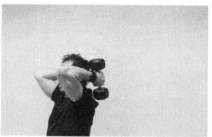

Pro-tip: Choose a lighter weight as this movement isolates only one joint, the triceps.

**Perpetuate: Shoulder presses:** *4 sets, 15 repetitions.*

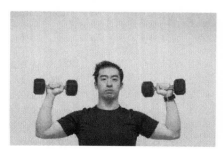 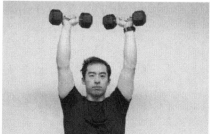

Pro-tip: You can choose a heavier weight for this movement.

## Perpetuate: Bear crawl: *4 sets, 45 seconds of crawl.*

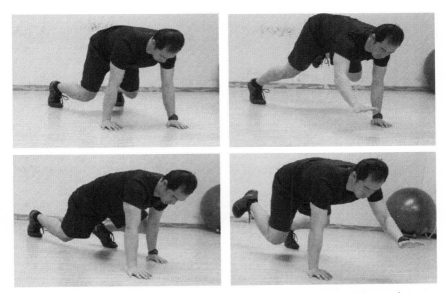

Pro-tip: Keep the back flat and the shoulders loaded on the elbow and wrist.

## Perpetuate: Bench dips: *4 sets, 10 repetitions.*

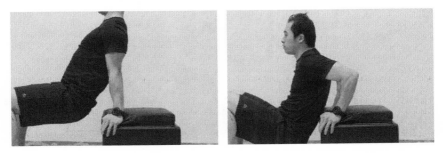

Pro-tip: Keep an upright posture and the elbows tucked inwards.

# Carpal Tunnel Syndrome

**Mobilize: Active range-of-motion - flexion, extension and deviations.** *2 sets, 10 repetitions each.*

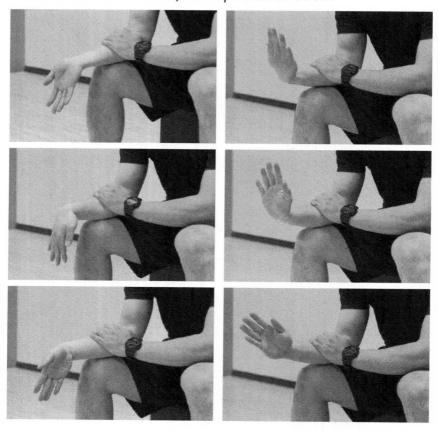

Pro-tip: Always go to full range-of-motion as long as pain allows it.

## Mobilize: Ulnar nerve floss: *2 sets, 10 repetitions per hand.*

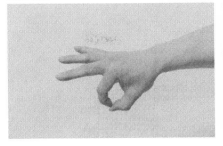 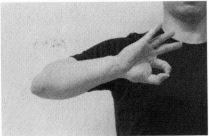

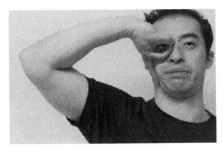

Pro-tip: Go as far as you feel a "nerve" stretch in the arm, then work your way to full range.

## Mobilize: Median nerve glide: *2 sets, 10 repetitions per arm.*

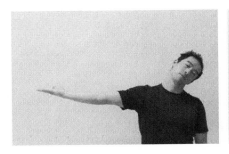 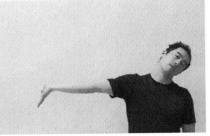

Pro-tip: Go as far as you feel a "nerve" stretch in the arm, then work your way to full range.

## Mobilize: Wrist band distraction: *2 sets, 10 repetition per arm.*

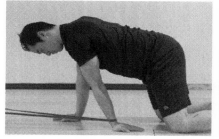 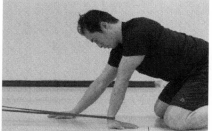

Pro-tip: Allow the band to pull your wrist forward while you move the arm back.

## Stabilize: Fist clenches: *3 sets, 10 repetitions.*

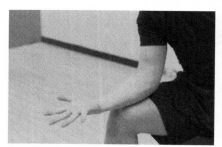 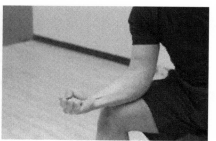

Pro-tip: Grip your fist as hard as you can then splay your hand as wide as you can.

## Strengthen: Grip strengthening: *3 sets, 45 seconds per arm.*

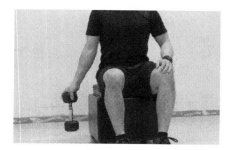

Pro-tip: Choose a weight that you can sustain the entire 45 seconds.

**Strengthen: Wall angels:** *4 sets, 15 repetitions.*

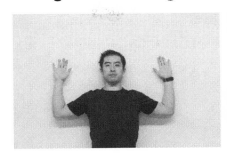 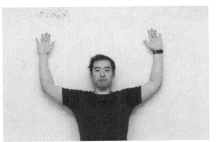

Pro-tip: Keep your elbows and wrists on the wall if you can.

**Strengthen: Dumbbell supinate + pronate:** *4 sets, 10 repetitions per hand.*

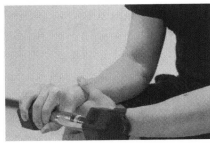 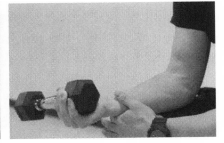

Pro-tip: Go to as much range-of-motion as pain will allow it.

**Strengthen: Band Ys:** *4 sets, 15 repetitions.*

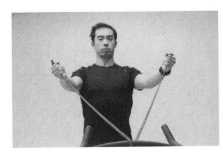 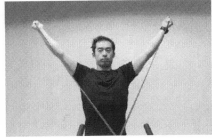

Pro-tip: Keep the shoulder blades peeled back and down. Squeeze the shoulder blades together during the entire movement.

**Perpetuate: High plank:** *4 sets, 1 minute.*

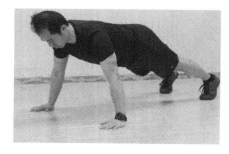

Pro-tip: Be aware of the pressure on the wrists. If you need to regress, put your knees down.

**Perpetuate: Renegade rows:** *4 sets, 10 repetitions per arm.*

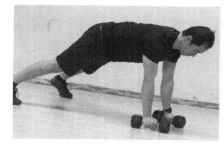 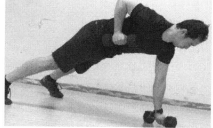

Pro-tip: Be aware of the pressure on the wrists. If you need to repress, put your knees down.

**Perpetuate: Push-ups:** *4 sets, 15 repetitions.*

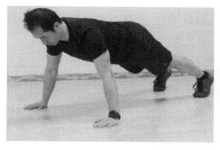 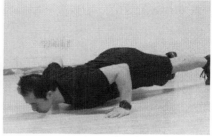

Pro-tip: There will be some pressure on your wrists. If you need to regress, put your knees down.

## Hand Fracture

**Mobilize: Lacrosse ball smash on forearms:** *2 sets, 45 seconds per side.*

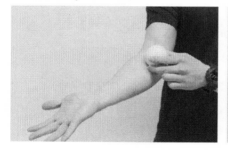 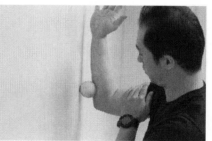

Pro-tip: Don't put the ball on any bony structures. Massage until area loosens up.

**Mobilize: Assisted wrist range-of-motion:** *2 sets, 10 repetitions per hand position.*

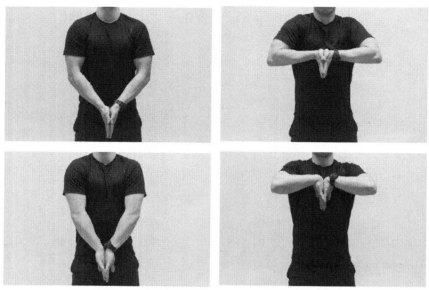

Pro-tip: Move through each repetitions in a fluid and controlled manner.

**Stabilize: 6 pack hand exercises:** *2 sets, 10 repetition per shape.*

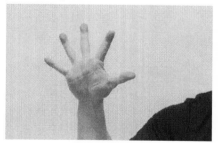 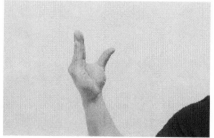

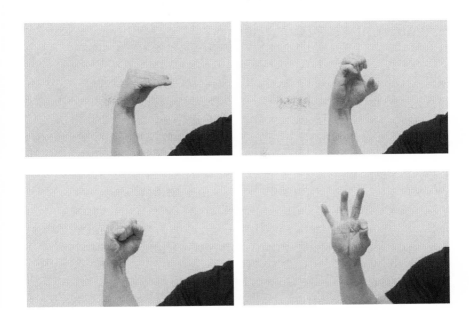

Pro-tip: Perform 10 repetition per hand shape for one set, then repeat for another. Each time a repetition is complete, return to open-splay hand.

## Stabilize: Wall finger push-ups: *3 sets, 10 repetitions.*

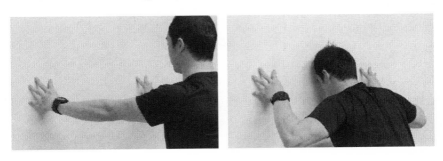

Pro-tip: Be aware of the pain levels in the hand through the movement. Keep the hand stiff.

### Strengthen: Grip-strengthening dumbbell holds: *3 sets, 45 seconds hold.*

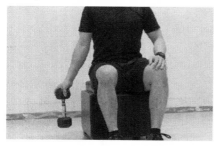

Pro-tip: Choose a weight that you can sustain for the entire 45 seconds.

### Strengthen: Towel wringing: *3 sets, 10 repetitions.*

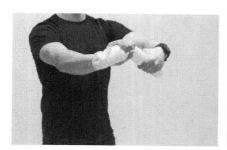 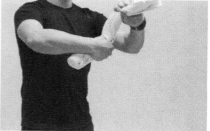

Pro-tip: Use full range-of-motion as far as pain will allow it.

### Strengthen: Dumbbell supinate + pronate: *4 sets, 10 repetitions.*

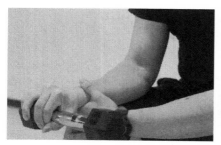 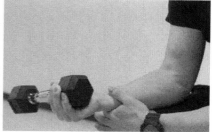

Pro-tip: Use full range-of-motion as far as pain will allow it.

## Strengthen: Wrist deviations with dowel: *4 sets, 10 repetitions.*

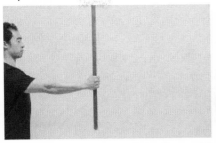 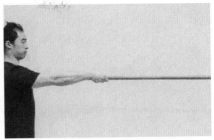

Pro-tip: Move through the entire movement in a controlled and fluid manner.

## Perpetuate: Overhead towel carries: *4 sets, 45 seconds walk.*

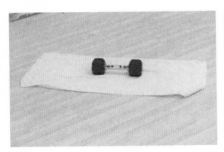 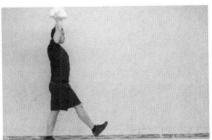

Pro-tip: Be aware of the pressure on the hand as you are holding the towel overhead.

## Perpetuate: Fist push-ups: *4 sets, 10 repetitions.*

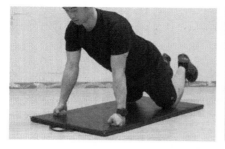 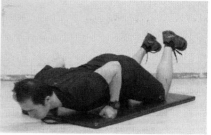

Pro-tip: Keep the wrist straight and as firm as possible.

## Perpetuate: Bear crawls: *4 sets, 45 seconds of crawl.*

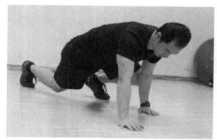 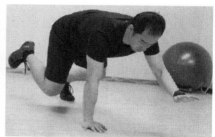

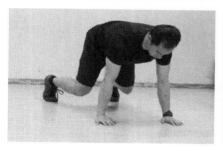 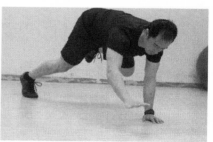

Pro-tip: Be aware of the pressure on the hand with each step.

# Finger Fracture

**Mobilize: Assisted finger range-of-motion:** *2 sets, 10 repetitions with the injured finger.*

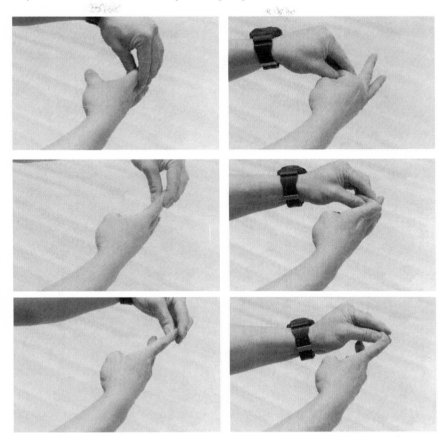

Pro-tip: Assist with injured finger through the range-of-motion that is tolerable.

**Stabilize: Fist + Claw:** *3 sets, 10 repetitions.*

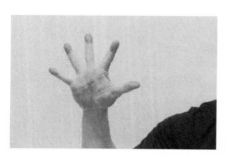 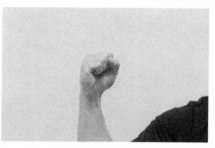 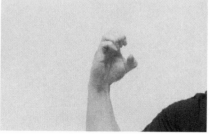

Pro-tip: Perform 10 repetition of hand to fist, then 10 repetitions of hand to claw, then repeat.

**Stabilize: Open hand wrist flexion + extension:** *3 sets, 10 repetitions.*

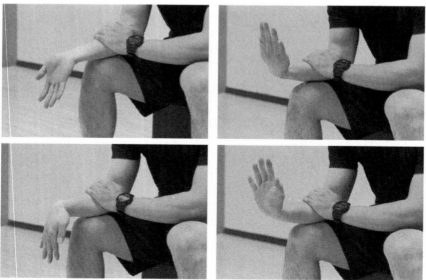

Pro-tip: Move through the tolerable full range-of-motion and keep movement controlled.

## Strengthen: Finger wall walks: 3 sets, 10 repetitions.

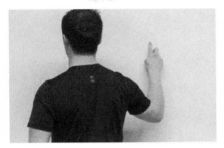
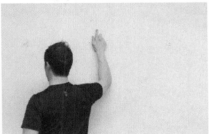

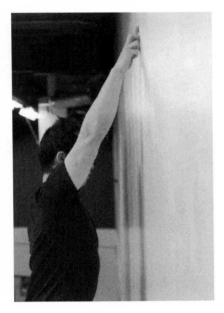

Pro-tip: Walk the fingers up the wall like a pair of legs. The idea is to get active movement into the finger.

**Strengthen: Farmer's carry:** *4 sets, 45 seconds of walk.*

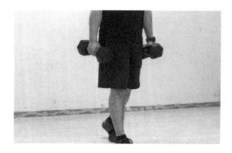

Pro-tip: Choose a weight that you can walk for the entire 45 seconds.

**Strengthen: Grip strengthening:** *4 sets, 45 seconds of hold.*

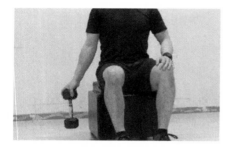

Pro-tip: Choose weight that you can sustain the entire 45 seconds.

**Strengthen: Wall finger push-ups:** *4 sets, 10 repetitions.*

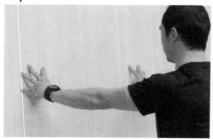 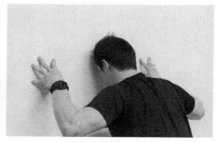

Pro-tip: Be mindful of the pressure that is put on the fingers.

## Perpetuate: Towel wrings: *4 sets, 10 repetitions.*

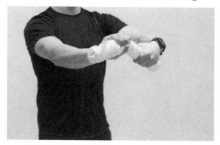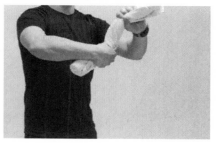

Pro-tip: Focus on the dynamic grip strength on the injured finger.

## Perpetuate: Fist push-ups: *4 sets, 10 repetitions.*

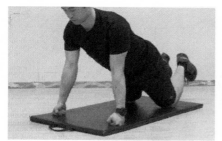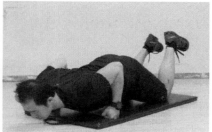

Pro-tip: Be aware of the pressure put on the finger inside the fist.

## Perpetuate: Towel carries: *4 sets, 45 seconds of walk.*

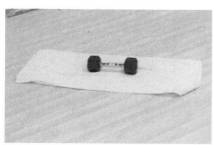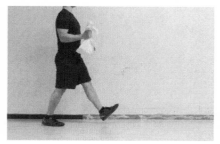

Pro-tip: Be aware of the pressure on the injured finger during the grip.

# Staple Stretches

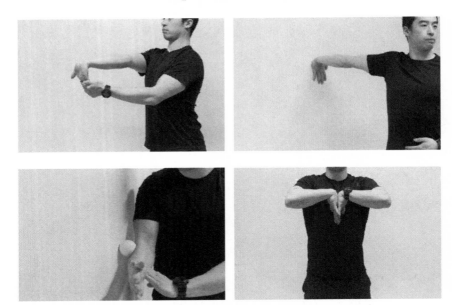

# 7. Lower back and hip injuries

Lower back can be most commonly known as **"lower cross syndrome"** and is simply a result of muscle strength imbalances in the trunk and lower body. These imbalances occur due to shortened or lengthened tissue in relation to each other.

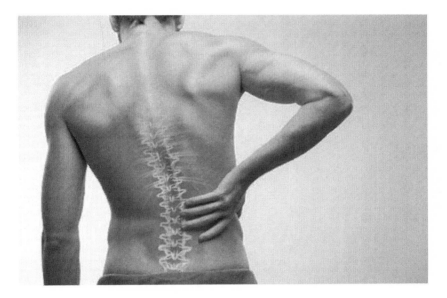

*eMedicineHealth (2019).*

**Back Stiff?**

Patients will often report tightness and/or pain in the lower back and hip flexors because of these imbalances. The hamstrings may also be reported as restricted. These imbalances collectively result in what's called an **anterior pelvic tilt**; or an excessive arch in the back during sitting or standing.

In my experience, individuals involved in a motor vehicle accident resulting from a "rear-ender" will most often report lower back pain. This is a soft tissue damage in the lower body which translates into the lower cross syndrome.

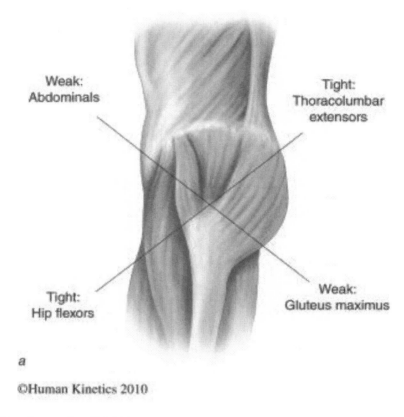

*Physio-pedia (2020).*

Treatment and rehabilitation

Treating these imbalances is simple and direct. Rehabilitation must target four of these areas and need to be performed daily to manage symptoms.

- **Glute strengthening.** The gluteal group is the largest muscle group in the body. Let's use it to our advantage. With lower cross syndrome, the gluteal group does not fire at the same efficiency relative to our entire body. In other words, if there is a strain or a load the lower back is under more strain compared to the glutes. This is what we DO NOT want. We want our glutes to do most of the work.

- **Core (abdominal) strengthening.** You often hear "lower back pain is a result of a "weak core". To some degree that is true but it isn't a definite factor. A weak core causes the pelvis to rotate anteriorly causing what's known as lumbar **lordosis**. It is an increased curvature in the lower back causing a compression in that region and ultimately leads to lower back pain. With core strengthening we can reverse the pelvic position and relieve the compression in the lumbar.

- **Hip flexor stretching.** Because the pelvis is rotated forward it causes stress and tension in the hip flexors. Often with lower back pain patients they will report lower back pain with tightness in the hips. Rehabilitation must also address the hip flexors as well. They may be tight, weak or both.

- **Lower back stretching.** In order to relieve tension in the low back, we can address it with various lower back stretches. Performing stretches will lengthen the tissues in the lumbar area as well as provide comfort for the patients with intense lower back pain. These stretches are recommended to be performed daily or even twice per day.

## Case about gluteus medius

The gluteus medius is often looked past because of the overbearing gluteus maximus. However, it has a very important role in hip health. It has been studied that strengthening the gluteus medius alongside with the gluteus maximus has shown high correlation with decreased lower back pain.

Because of origin and insertion point of the gluteus medius, it has a significant effect on hip health. Strengthening the gluteus medius it will increase the stability in the pelvic-sacral region as well as the relationship between the femur and pelvis. More stability is never a bad thing; given that we have full range of motion in the joint.

The more firing of the gluteal group we can get, the more strain we can take out of the lumbar region so work on that butt!

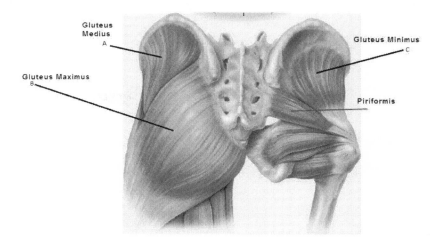

*Sastre (2019).*

## Daily habits and lifestyle changes

In order for lower back pain to have the lowest impact on everyday life, several changes must occur.

### 1.) Walk more and often

- This activity is a low-risk, high-reward type of activity. It can be done anywhere and anyone can do it. Every structure in the human body is connected in some way. Walk! Move around! Move at a pace fast enough so it allows you to swing your arms. Any type of movement is beneficial to the low back. Start out small, like walking around the block, then build from there. If you experience pain with walking, you are probably doing too much and too fast.

### 2.) Stand up at least once per hour

- Too much of anything is not good. In other words, too much sitting is not good. Break the sitting schedule with a standing break. It doesn't need to be long; just five to 10 minutes will do. Standing will reset the trunk and hips into a more natural "extension", which is something positive for the low back.

### 3.) Check your sitting posture

- Every hour there should be a self-check on your sitting posture. This is too make sure that you are not slouched over. And if you are, this is your chance to correct it before the next hour.

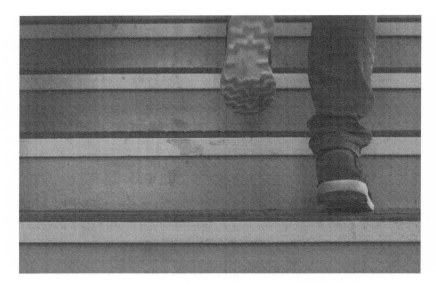

*Hills (2014).*

### Middle Back Pain?

T-spine, also known as thoracic spine, is the second "section" of the spinal cord under the C-spine (cervical). It begins at the shoulders and ends where the lower back begins (of course this is an approximation). Patients with middle back pain with report pain symptoms around this area.

To treat middle back pain we must target two issues: thoracic mobility and serratus anterior stability.

1.) Patients that report middle back pain will almost always show a restricted T-spine. With decreased mobility in this area it will cause complications with the middle back, shoulders and lower back.

The movement of the T-spine is quite versatile. It can bend forward, backward, side-flex and rotate. Our goal is to restore the movement in the T-spine. We can restore flexion and extension by putting a foam roller underneath the shoulder blades and moving through flexion and extension. This will allow the foam roller to act as wedge in the middle of our T-spine while the top-portion extends and "opens up". Remember to keep your core area braced as you move through the movement.

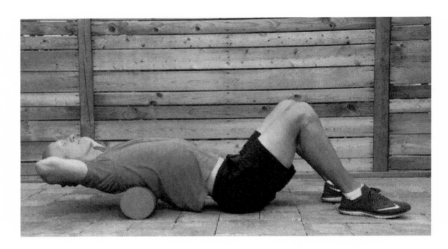

*Westcoast SCI (2018).*

Rotation is another key pattern of the thoracic spine. For patients who have lower back pain, it is recommended to prescribe more T-spine rotation movements. Using the open-book exercise, it will allow us to work on rotation of the T-spine. It is key to keep your hips and legs frozen as we move through the movement with our upper body. This will isolate the T-spine and allow it to work through the range and restore the mobility.

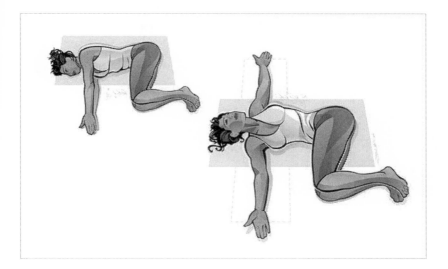

*Grauer (2016).*

2.) Serratus Anterior Stability

If you look at the relationship between the serratus anterior muscle and the middle back, they are closely related. This muscle begins at the outside surface of the upper eight or nine ribs and connects to the middle border other scapula. It holds the scapula in place to the chest wall.

The take-away point is this: because the attachment point is in the middle back, as long as we strengthen the serratus we are able to counterbalance out symptoms in the middle back. In other words, middle back and the rib cage are opposites. The serratus anterior muscle is the connector. To take the strain off the middle back, we thus train the serratus.

There are numerous ways to train the serratus. One of my favourite is the push-ups plus. Remember that this muscle holds the scapula in place and counterbalances in the middle back.

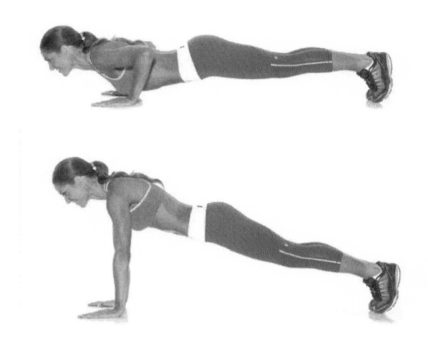

*Calderone (2019).*

## Pain in the "SI joint"

Patients with lower back injuries often report muscle stiffness and discomfort. They are referring to the "softer" part of the back muscles. However, some patients may refer to a more "hip" type pain and occurs slightly lower than the middle back; less of a muscle stiffness and more of a joint pain.

This joint connects both the hip bones onto the sacrum (the structure between the spine and the tailbone). The main function of this "SI" joint is to absorb shock between the upper body and the legs. There is very little movement at this joint and is reinforced by strong ligaments around it. There is a system of soft tissues at this joint to help absorb shock and to provide support. Other supporting muscles include the gluteal group and the piriformis.

It is more tricky to treat SI joint issues because it is more difficult to "get to" because it's a joint and to treat it we must target the muscles surrounding it. Often with hip issues I like to prescribe CARs – controlled articular rotations. The keyword is controlled. When the hip is moving around the joint, in a controlled fashion, the muscles must be engaged and activated in order for the leg to come around. When we require the body to the motionless while the leg is moving, stabilizers must also engage to keep the body and joints "stacked". Thus, to target the SI joint (or the stabilizers) we must force our body to use those stabilizers.

## Treatments

# Lower Back Pain (Lower Cross Syndrome)

**Mobilize: Cat-cows:** *2 sets, 10 repetitions.*

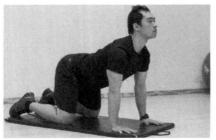 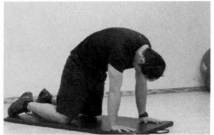

Pro-tip: Look up with the eyes then look down as far as you can on the down portion.

**Mobilize: Window wipers:** *2 sets, 10 repetitions per side.*

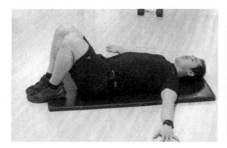 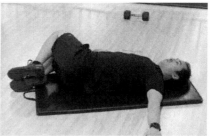

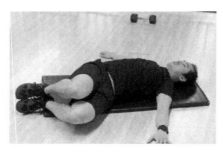

Pro-tip: Keep your shoulders from lifting off the ground during the entire movement.

### Mobilize: Prone press-ups: *2 sets, 10 repetitions.*

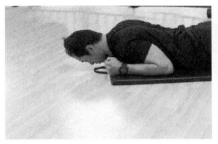 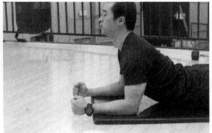

Pro-tip: Go as far as you need to feel the stretch. To progress, go on your hands.

### Stabilize: Plank: *2 sets, 45 seconds of hold.*

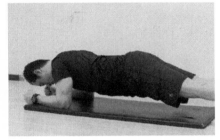

Pro-tip: Curl the hips inwards so that you don't arch your back. This will engage the core area.

### Stabilize: Glute bridges: *3 sets, 15 repetitions.*

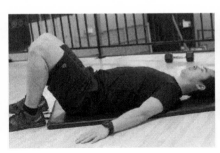 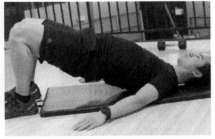

Pro-tip: Drive the hips up from the heels and squeeze the butt-cheeks at the top.

**Stabilize: Partial curl-ups:** *3 sets, 10 repetitions.*

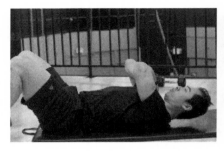 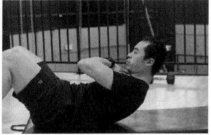

Pro-tip: Keep the chin tucked in and curl right as the shoulder blades leave the floor.

**Strengthen: Bird-dogs:** *4 sets, 10 repetitions per side.*

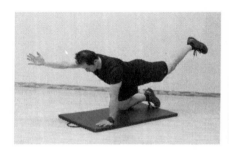 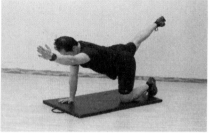

Pro-tip: Keep the chin tucked in. Lift at the hips and the shoulders.

**Strengthen: Palloff presses:** *4 sets, 10 repetitions per side.*

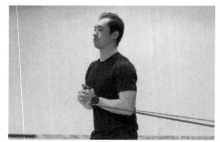 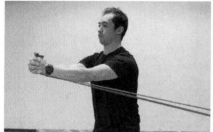

Pro-tip: Line yourself up so that the band is coming in from the side. Push the band directly in front of you.

### Strengthen: Bent-leg lifts: *4 sets, 20 repetitions.*

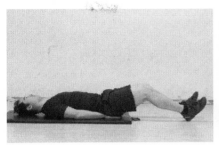 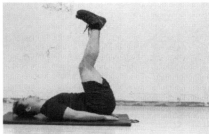

Pro-tip: The hands are placed underneath the hips to support the lower back. Press your abdominals downwards to engage the core area.

### Strengthen: Goblet squats: *4 sets, 15 repetitions.*

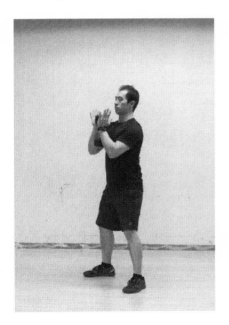 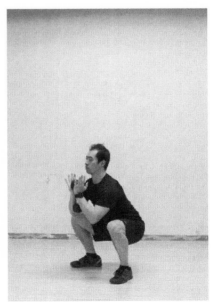

Pro-tip: Push the hips back and drive the knees outwards.

**Perpetuate: Supermans:** *4 sets, 10 repetitions.*

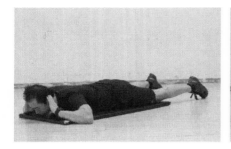 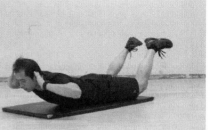

Pro-tip: Squeeze the butt-cheeks before you lift the torso and legs.

**Perpetuate: Swiss ball roll-out:** *4 sets, 10 repetitions.*

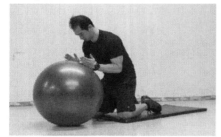 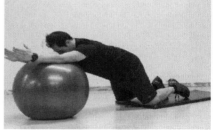

Pro-tip: Keep the chin tucked in as you roll the ball forward. Keep the torso stiff.

**Perpetuate: Barbell deadlifts: 4 sets, 10 repetitions.**

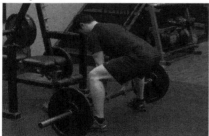 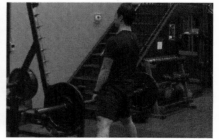

Pro-tip: Keep the back straight and lift with the legs while keeping the torso stiff.

# Middle Back Pain

**Mobilize: Foam-roller body openers:** *2 sets, 10 repetitions.*

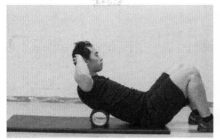 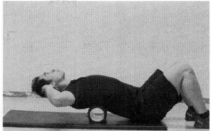

Pro-tip: Place the foam roller underneath the shoulder blades and arch slowly.

**Mobilize: Half-kneeling body openers:** *2 sets, 10 repetitions per leg.*

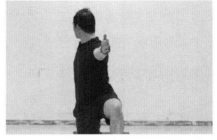

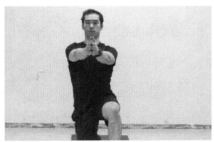

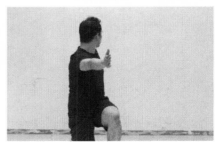

Pro-tip: Both left and right hand is one repetition. Remember to change legs for a complete set.

**Stabilize: Quadraped rotating reaches:** *2 sets, 10 repetitions per arm.*

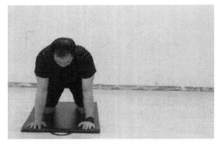 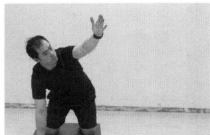

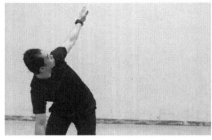

Pro-tip: You are making a "backstroke" movement. Rotate the body as much as possible.

**Stabilize: Scapulae push-up:** *3 sets, 10 repetitions.*

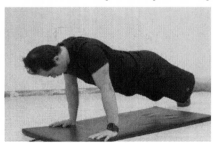 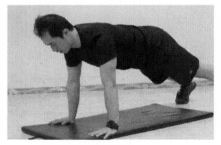

Pro-tip: The movement is in the shoulder blades moving in and out.

## Strengthen: Y press-outs: *4 sets, 15 repetitions.*

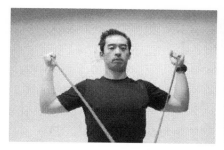 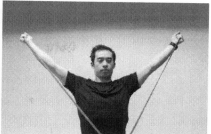

Pro-tip: Keep the shoulders peeled back and lock the arms out at the top.

## Strengthen: Push-up plus: *4 sets, 10 repetitions.*

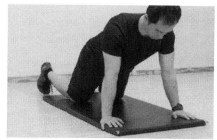 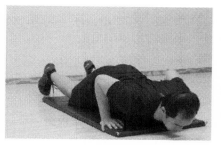

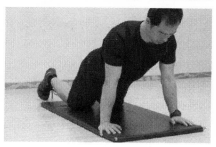 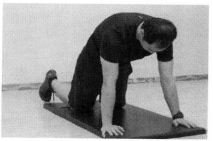

Pro-tip: First do the push-up, then cave the chest in at the top. You are targeting the serratus anterior muscle.

**Strengthen: Band punch reaches:** *4 sets, 15 repetitions per side.*

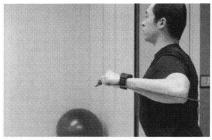
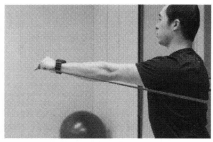
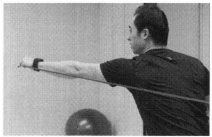

Pro-tip: You must focus on the reach (last image) after the punch.

**Strengthen: Side bridges:** *4 sets, 10 repetitions per side.*

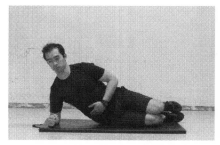
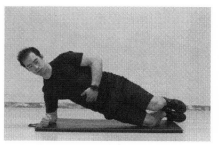

Pro-tip: Keep the trunk and shoulder stiff as you lift the hips up.

**Perpetuate: Underarm pull-downs:** *4 sets, 15 repetitions.*

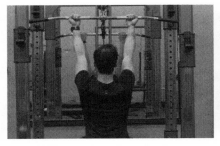 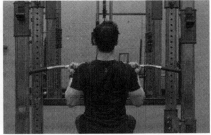

Pro-tip: Keep the shoulders back and down as you pull down on the bar.

**Perpetuate: Band woodchoppers:** *4 sets, 10 repetitions per side.*

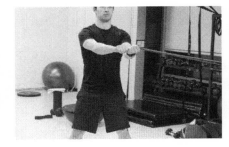 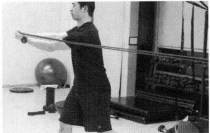

Pro-tip: Rotate the trunk as you pull the band.

**Perpetuate: Back hyperextensions:** *4 sets, 10 repetitions.*

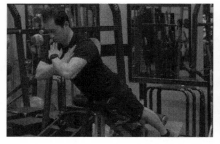 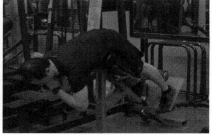

Pro-tip: Engage the glutes before you pull body upwards.

# Hip Fracture

**Mobilize: Hip controlled articular rotations:** *2 sets, 5 repetitions per side.*

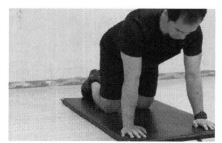 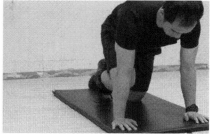

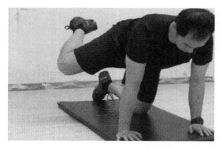 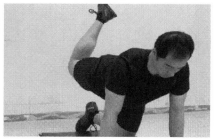

Pro-tip: Aim for 5 seconds per rotation.

## Mobilize: Groiners: *2 sets, 5 repetitions per side.*

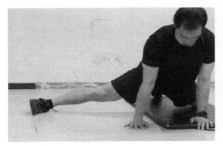 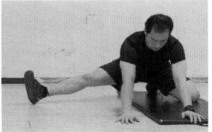

Pro-tip: Point the toe on the straight leg upwards as you rock the hips back.

## Mobilize: Hip crosses: 2 sets, 5 repetitions.

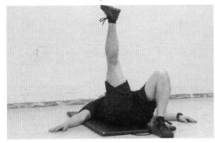 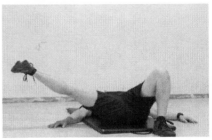

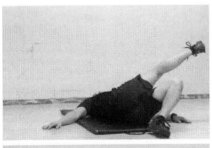 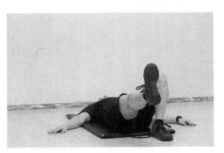

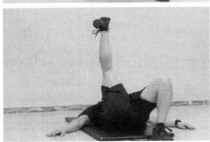

Pro-tip: Move through the range slowly, making a cross. Each time a cross is made is one repetition.

**Stabilize: Single leg balance:** *3 sets, 45 seconds of hold.*

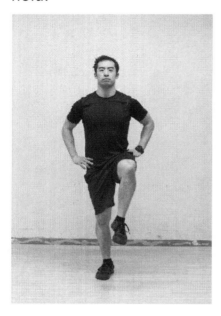

Pro-tip: Keep the standing leg stiff and hips balanced throughout. To progress, close your eyes.

**Stabilize: Bird-dog:** *3 sets, 10 repetitions per side.*

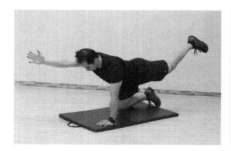 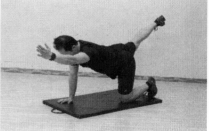

Pro-tip: Lift with your hips and shoulders.

**Stabilize: Side-lying hip abductions:** *3 sets, 10 repetitions per side.*

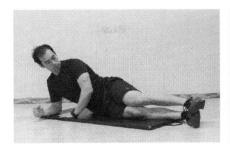 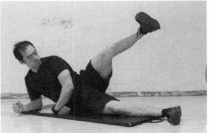

Pro-tip: Lift at the hip and keep the toes pointing forward.

**Strengthen: Band hip-flexor strengthening:** *4 sets, 15 repetitions per side.*

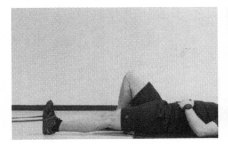 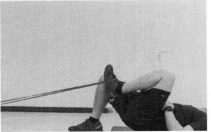

Pro-tip: Drive the knees towards the chest.

**Strengthen: Glute bridges:** *4 sets, 15 repetitions.*

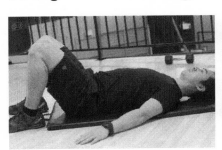 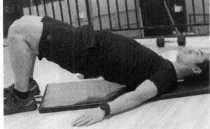

Pro-tip: Drive from the heels and clench the butt-cheeks at the top of the movement.

**Strengthen: Superclams:** *4 sets, 10 repetitions per side.*

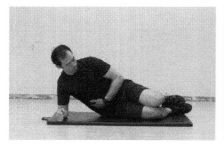 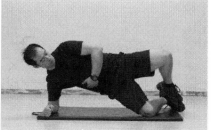

Pro-tip: Lift the hips and open the knee at the same time.

**Strengthen: Single-leg quarter squats:** *4 sets, 10 repetitions per side.*

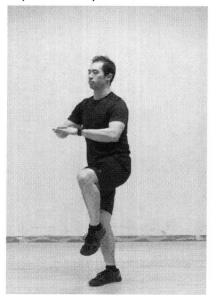 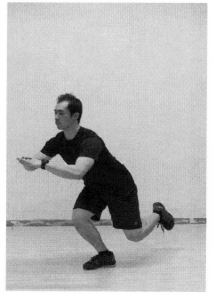

Pro-tip: Push the hips back and slightly lean forward with the body.

**Perpetuate: Lateral lunges:** *4 sets, 5 repetitions per side.*

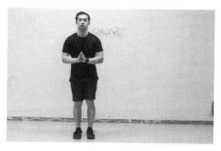 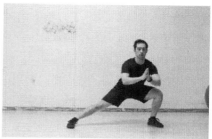

Pro-tip: Lunge as wide and as deep as pain will allow. Add weight for progression.

**Perpetuate: Low-and-Slow:** *4 sets, 10 repetitions.*

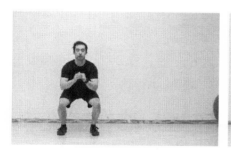 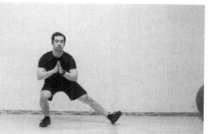

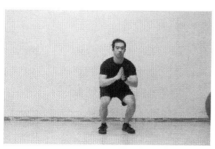

Pro-tip: Keep the head at the same height during the entire set.

**Perpetuate: Goblet squats:** *4 sets, 15 repetitions.*

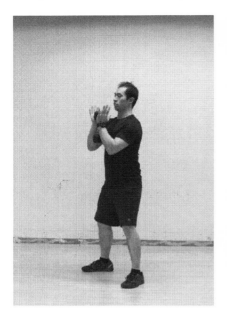 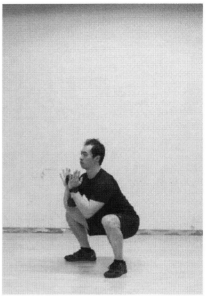

Pro-tip: Push the hips back and go as deep as pain would allow it,

# Hip Flexor Strain

**Mobilize: Foam roll hip flexor + quadriceps:** *2 sets, 45 seconds per area per side.*

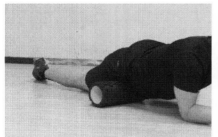 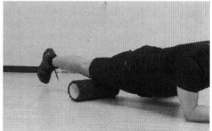

Pro-tip: Work on the hip flexor first for 45 seconds, then move down to the quads for 45 seconds. Find a tender spot and allow the body weight to sink in.

**Mobilize: Dynamic hip flexor stretch:** *2 sets, 5 per side.*

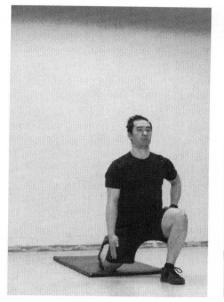 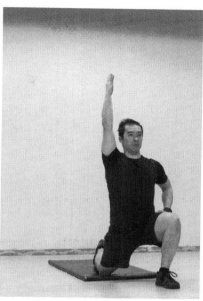

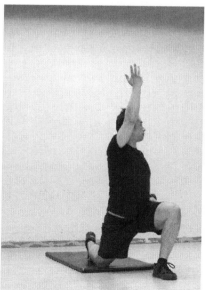

Pro-tip: Keep the movement fluid and controlled. Move through the full range-of-motion.

**Stabilize: Seated heel slides:** *3 sets, 10 repetitions per side.*

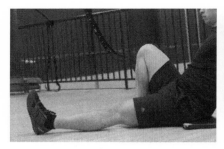 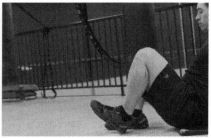

Pro-tip: Pull the foot in by squeezing the hamstrings.

**Stabilize: Clam shells:** *3 sets, 20 repetitions per side.*

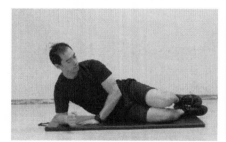 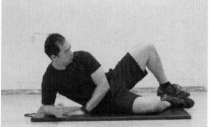

Pro-tip: You are working on the hips as you open the knees.

**Stabilize: Single-leg glute bridges:** *3 sets, 10 repetitions per side.*

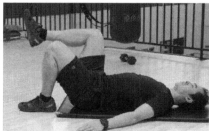 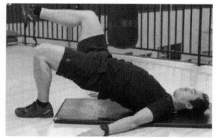

Pro-tip: Drive the hips up using the heel and squeeze the butt cheek at the top.

## Strengthen: Standing band hip flexion: *4 sets, 10 repetitions per side.*

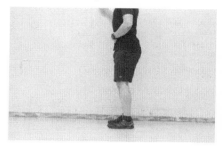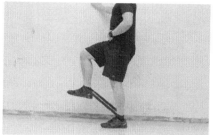

Pro-tip: Stand tall during the entire movement and lift the leg using the hip.

## Strengthen: Assisted sumo squats: *4 sets, 15 repetitions.*

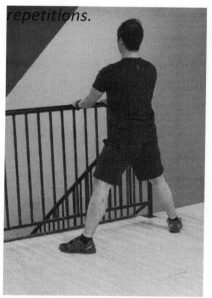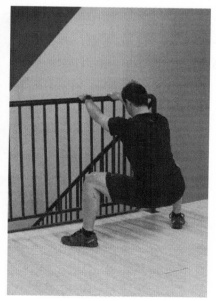

Pro-tip: Push the knees out as far as you can. For progression, do it unassisted.

**Strengthen: Wall sits:** *4 sets, 45 seconds of hold.*

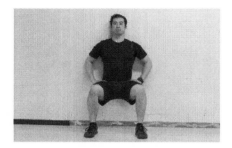

Pro-tip: Push your knees out and sit until thighs are parallel.

## Strengthen: Slow tempo mountain climbers: *4 sets, 10 repetitions per side.*

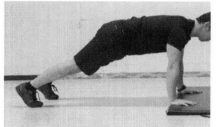 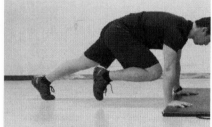

Pro-tip: This is a slow movement. Aim for 2 seconds per repetition.

## Perpetuate: Step-ups: *4 sets, 10 repetitions per side.*

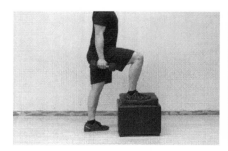 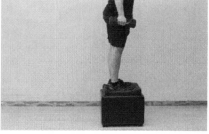

Pro-tip: Drive the body up at the heel and stand straight up at the top.

**Perpetuate: Leg lifts:** *4 sets, 20 repetitions.*

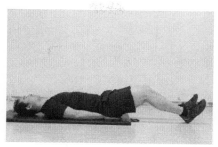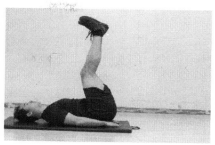

Pro-tip: Keep the leg slightly bent and push the abdominals downwards.

**Perpetuate: Lunges:** *4 sets, 10 repetitions per leg.*

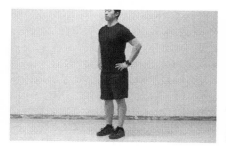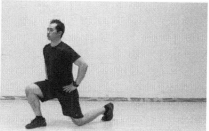

Pro-tip: Keep the body upright as you lunge down.

# Hip Flexor Strain

**Mobilize: Leg swings - forward + lateral:** *2 sets, 5 repetitions each direction.*

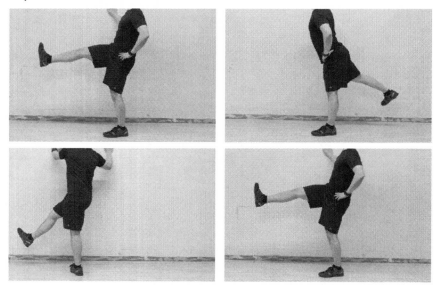

Pro-tip: Swings are controlled and should provide a very slight stretch.

**Mobilize: Dynamic figure 4:** *2 sets, 5 repetitions per side.*

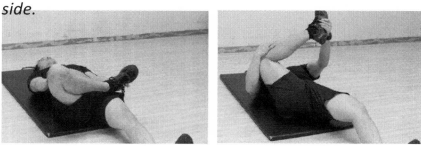

Pro-tip: Guide the leg slowly up and down while maintaining the 90-90 at the hip and knee.

**Stabilize: Standing hip openers:** *3 sets, 5 repetitions per side.*

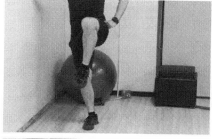 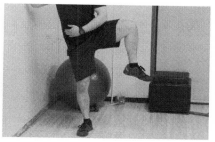

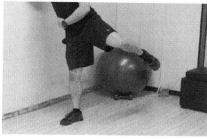

Pro-tip: All 3 steps are performed very controlled. Twist the heel as high as possible in the last step.

**Stabilize: Standing kick-backs:** *3 sets, 10 repetitions per leg.*

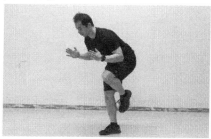 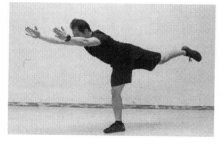

Pro-tip: Reach and kick out at the same time; challenging your core and structural stability.

**Stabilize: Quarter single leg squats:** *3 sets, 10 repetitions per leg.*

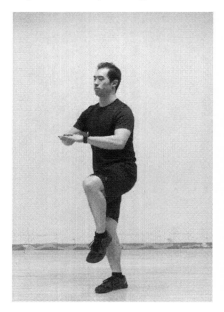 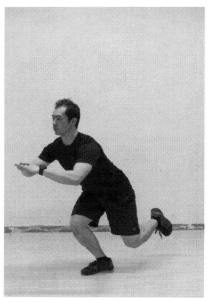

Pro-tip: The body can lean forward slightly as you bend down.

**Strengthen: Bird-dogs:** *4 sets, 10 repetitions per side.*

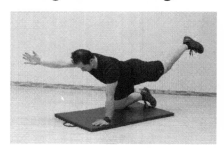 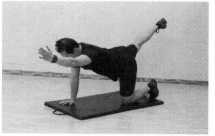

Pro-tip: Lift at the heel and the shoulder. Keep the torso rigid during the movement.

**Strengthen: Reverse Nordic curls:** *4 sets, 10 repetitions.*

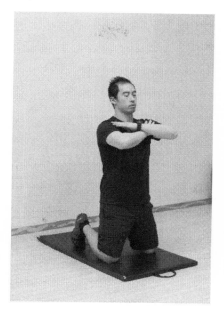 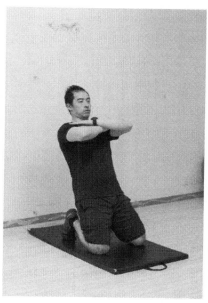

Pro-tip: Keep the hips pushed forward during the entire movement. Aim for a 3 second count.

**Strengthen: Big swimmers:** *4 sets, 20 repetitions per side.*

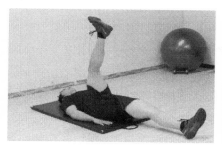 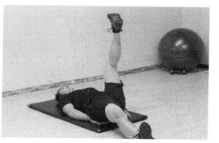

Pro-tip: The hands are under the hips to support the lower back. This is working on the endurance of the hip flexors.

**Strengthen: Sumo squats:** *4 sets, 15 repetitions.*

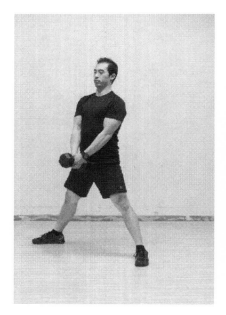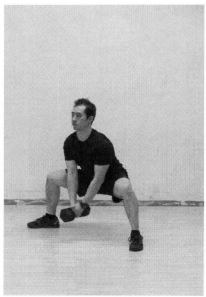

Pro-tip: Push the knees out as far as you can. You can choose a heavier weight if you prefer.

**Perpetuate: Curtsy squats:** *4 sets, 10 repetitions per side.*

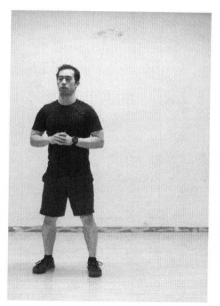 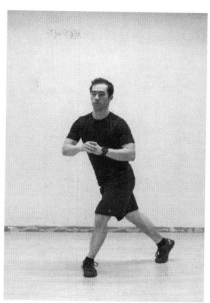

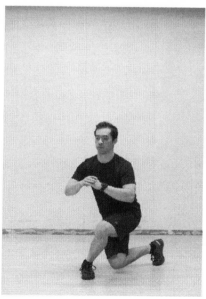

Pro-tip: Step diagonal to about 45 degrees. Keep the torso upright when squatting.

**Perpetuate: Mountain climber + kick-out:** *4 sets, 10 repetitions per side.*

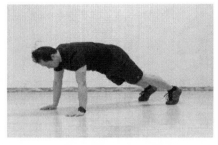 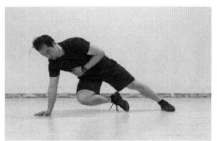

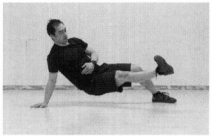

Pro-tip: Keep the shoulder stiff when you kick out in the last step.

**Perpetuate: Rear foot elevated squats:** *4 sets, 10 repetitions per side.*

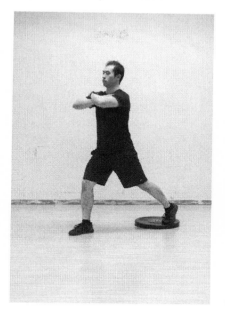 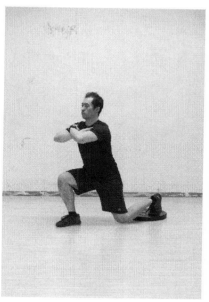

Pro-tip: Keep the body upright during the entire movement. Use weights to progress.

# Labral Tear in the Hip

**Mobilize: Hip flexor flow:** *2 sets, 5 repetitions per side.*

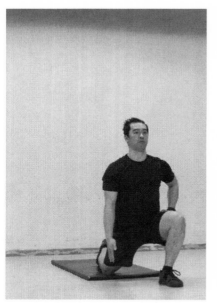 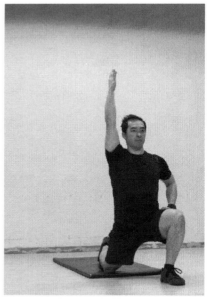

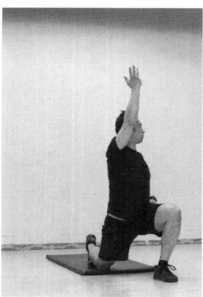

Pro-tip: Do each step in a controlled and fluid fashion.

## **Mobilize: Standing hip openers:** *2 sets, 5 repetitions per leg.*

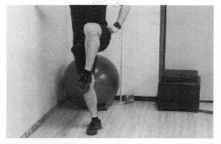 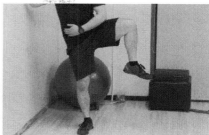

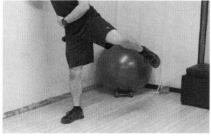

Pro-tip: Aim for second per movement.

## **Mobilize: Sitting groin openers:** *2 sets, 10 repetitions.*

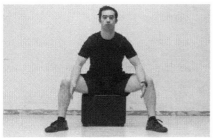 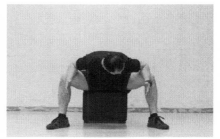

Pro-tip: Slowly push the knees apart with the forearms. Feel the stretch in the groin area.

**Stabilize: Single bent-leg balance:** *3 sets, 30 seconds of hold.*

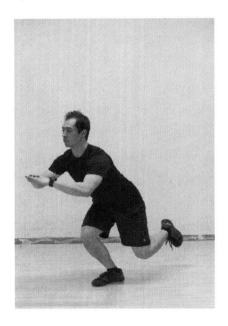

Pro-tip: Push the hips back and bend the knee slightly.

**Stabilize: Bosu ball balance:** *3 sets, 45 seconds of hold.*

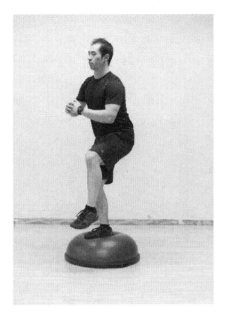

Pro-tip: Keep a slight bend in the standing leg.

**Stabilize: Swiss ball hamstring curls:** *3 sets, 10 repetitions.*

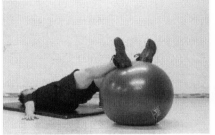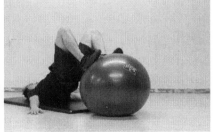

Pro-tip: Keep the hips lifted and pull the ball in with the heels.

**Strengthen: Feet on Swiss ball plank:** *4 sets, 1 minute holds.*

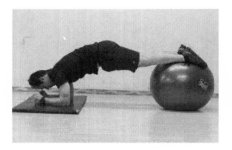

Pro-tip: Keep the hips "rolled in" so that the core engages.

**Strengthen: Frog pump:** *4 sets, 20 repetitions.*

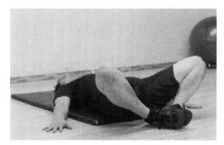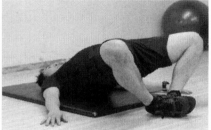

Pro-tip: Keep the heels together and use the heels to drive the hips up.

**Strengthen: Low + Slow:** *4 sets, 10 repetitions.*

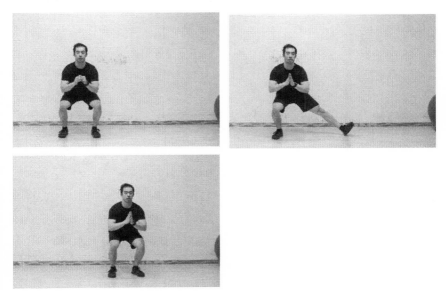

Pro-tip: Keep the head level the same throughout the entire set.

**Strengthen: Rear-leg elevated squats:** *4 sets, 10 repetitions per leg.*

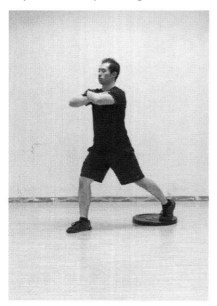 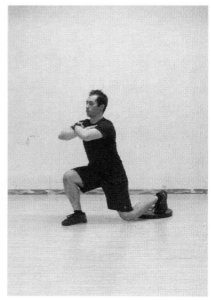

Pro-tip: Bend the back leg while keeping the torso upright. The front leg will bend automatically.

**Perpetuate: Reverse hyper extensions:** *4 sets, 10 repetitions.*

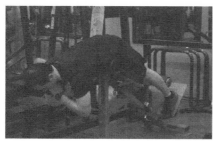 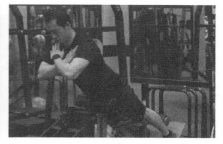

Pro-tip: Squeeze the glutes before pulling the upper body up.

**Perpetuate: Single-leg deadlifts:** *4 sets, 10 repetitions per leg.*

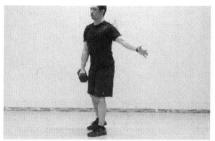 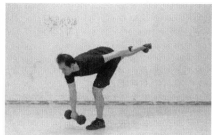

Pro-tip: Keep a slight bend in the standing leg when you hinge the body.

**Perpetuate: Rocket jumps:** *4 sets, 5 repetitions.*

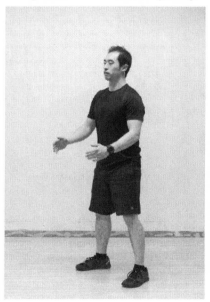 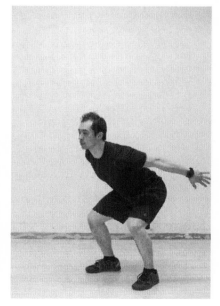

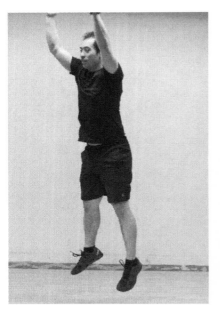
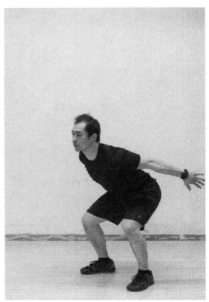

Pro-tip: Land in an "athletic position" meaning knees slightly bend and chest out.

---

# Sciatica (Piriformis Syndrome)

**Mobilize: Foam rolling piriformis, IT band +**
**hamstrings:** *2 sets, 45 seconds each.*

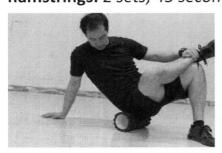
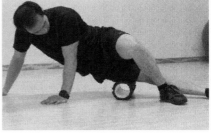

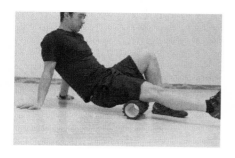

Pro-tip: Roll until you find a "sore spot" then put your weight into that spot to release it.

## Mobilize: Nerve glide: *2 sets, 10 repetitions.*

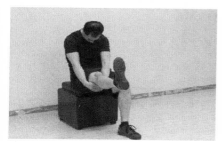 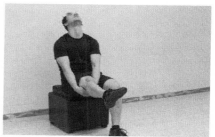

Pro-tip: The point of this is to loosen up the nerve that runs down the leg.

## Mobilize: Nerve floss: *2 sets, 10 repetitions.*

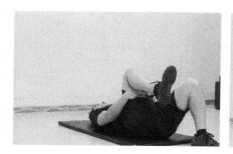 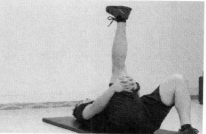

Pro-tip: Straighten the leg as far as you can until a stretch is felt.

**Mobilize: Dynamic figure 4:** *2 sets, 10 repetitions.*

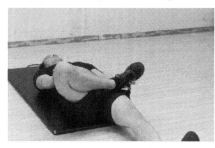 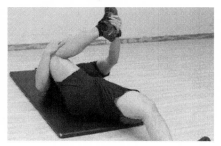

Pro-tip: Keep the figure 4 shape as you move the leg up and down.

**Stabilize: Clam shells:** *3 sets, 20 repetitions per side.*

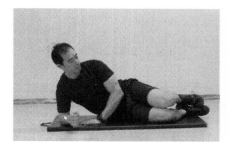 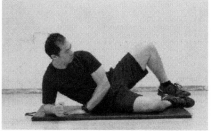

Pro-tip: Use the hip muscles to peel the knee open.

**Stabilize: Bench glute bridges:** *3 sets, 10 repetitions.*

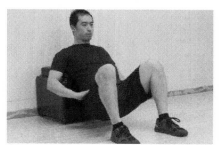 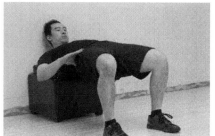

Pro-tip: Keep the chin tucked downwards as the hips come up to prevent any neck injuries.

**Strengthen: Prone hip extension:** *4 sets, 10 repetitions per side.*

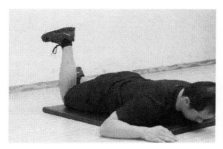 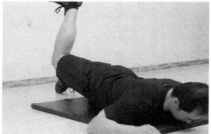

Pro-tip: Keep the hips on the floor as much as possible.

**Strengthen: Supermans:** *4 sets, 10 repetitions.*

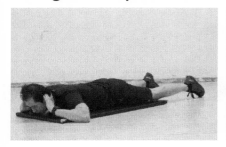 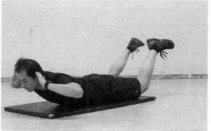

Pro-tip: Squeeze the butt cheeks before lifting the legs and torso.

### Strengthen: Standing hip abduction: *4 sets, 20 repetitions per side.*

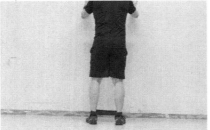 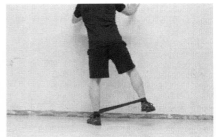

Pro-tip: Keep standing tall and keep the toes pointed forward.

### Strengthen: Bodyweight hip-hinges: *4 sets, 10 repetitions per side.*

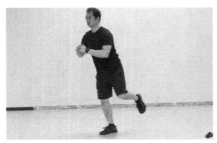 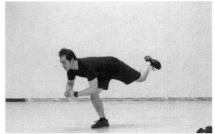

Pro-tip: Keep the back straight and keep a slight bend in the standing leg.

### Perpetuate: Lateral lunges: *4 sets, 10 repetitions per side.*

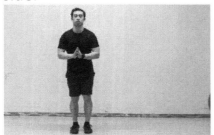 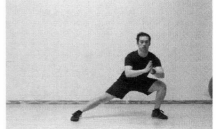

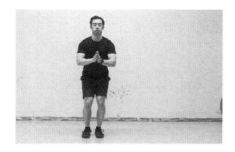

Pro-tip: Push the knee out to the side as you step into the lunge.

## Perpetuate: Single hamstring curls: *4 sets, 10 repetitions per side.*

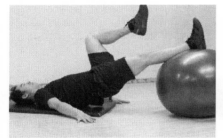 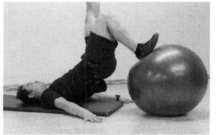

Pro-tip: Keep the hips up as you curl the ball in and as you straighten your leg.

**Perpetuate: Curtsy lunges:** *4 sets, 10 repetitions per side.*

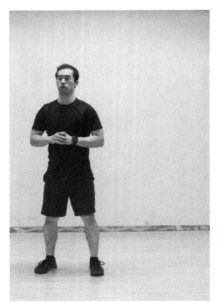
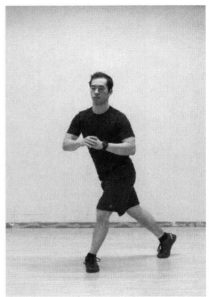
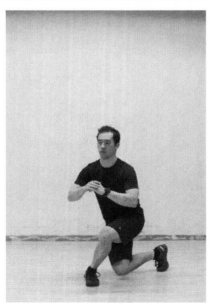

Pro-tip: Step diagonal at about 45 degrees before you squat down.

# SI Joint Pain

## Mobilize: Prone single-leg internal + external rotation: *2 sets, 10 repetitions per leg*

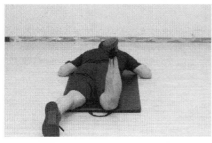 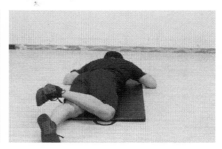

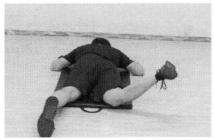

Pro-tip: Rotate the leg only at the hip joint.

## Mobilize: Fire hydrants: *2 sets, 10 rotations per leg.*

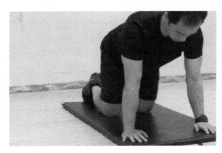 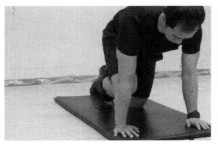

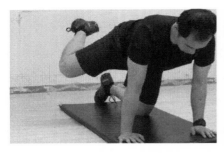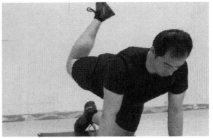

Pro-tip: Keep the hips flat. Draw circles with the knee.

## Mobilize: Hip shin-box transfers: *2 sets, 10 repetitions.*

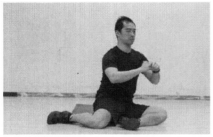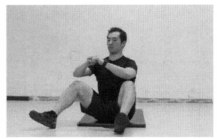

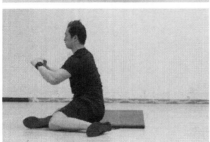

Pro-tip: Keep the body upright. Ensure the knees and heels touch the floor per transfer.

### Stabilize: Squat holds: *3 sets, 45 second holds.*

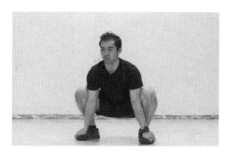

Pro-tip: Keep the body upright and push the knees out with your arms.

### Stabilize: Band lateral toe-taps: *3 sets, 15 per leg.*

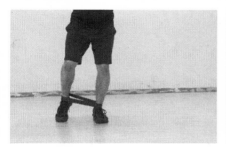 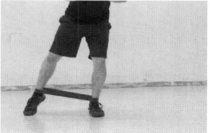

Pro-tip: Keep a slight bend in the standing leg and keep the body from moving.

### Strengthen: Ball squeeze glute bridges: *4 sets, 20 repetitions.*

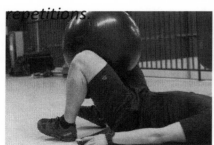 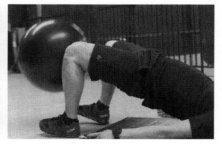

Pro-tip: You can substitute the Swiss ball for another type of ball (ie. Basketball).

### Strengthen: Super clams: *4 sets, 10 repetitions per side.*

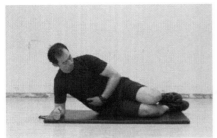 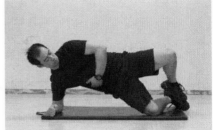

Pro-tip: Push the hips up and open the knees at the same time.

### Strengthen: Band glute bridges: *4 sets, 20 repetitions.*

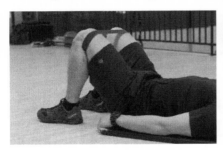 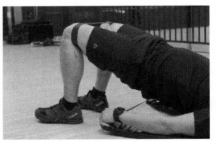

Pro-tip: Drive the knees out before pushing the hips up.

## Strengthen: Superman: *4 sets, 15 repetitions.*

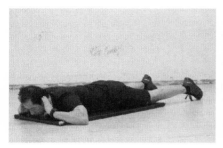 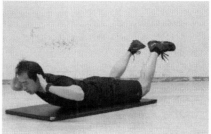

Pro-tip: Squeeze the butt-cheeks before lifting the body and legs.

## Perpetuate: Lateral lunge weight-shifts: *4 sets, 10 per side.*

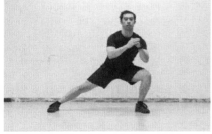 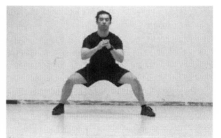

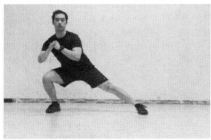

Pro-tip: Push the knees out and keep the head the same level.

**Perpetuate: Rear foot elevated squats:** *4 sets, 10 repetitions per side.*

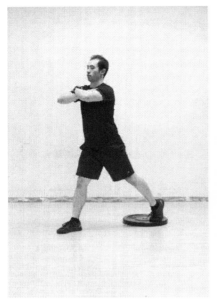 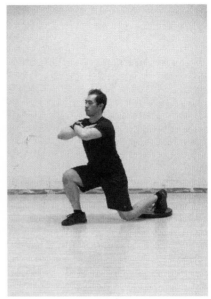

Pro-tip: Drop the back leg; the front will bend automatically.

**Perpetuate: Bound and absorb:** *4 sets, 5 repetitions per leg.*

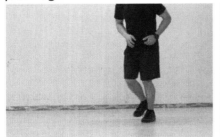 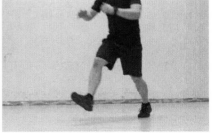

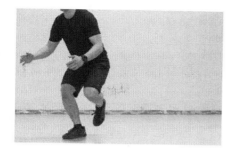

Pro-tip: Land with the leg bent in an athletic position.

# Staple Stretches

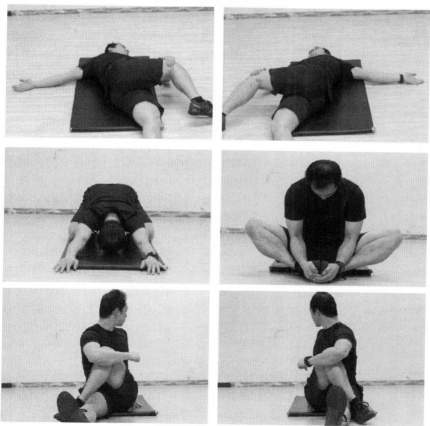

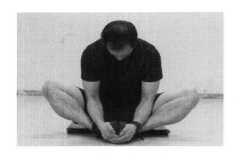

# **8.** Leg and knee injuries

**Knee Science**

Although your knee is responsible of a single-joint movement (it only flexes and extends), it has a lot of complicated components making it vulnerable to various injuries. Some of these include fractures, dislocations, sprains, ligament tears and simply wear and tear. At the extreme end, some injuries require surgery to correct.

The knee is the one of the most complex joint in the body and connects the femur, tibia, fibula and the knee cap. It contains fluid inside the capsule making it a synovial joint.

Various ligaments of the knee connect to bind bony structures together. These bands of white, fibrous and slightly elastic tissue prevent dislocation and restrict excessive movement to the knee. These ligaments include the iliotibial band (ITB), anterior cruciate ligament (ACL), posterior cruciate ligament (PCL), medial collateral ligament (MCL) and the lateral collateral ligament (LCL).

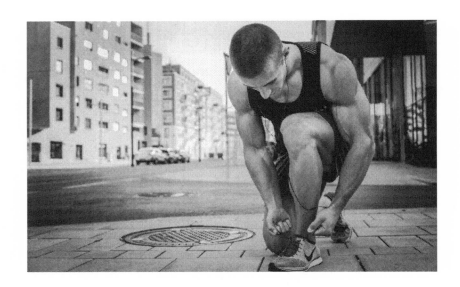

*Redl (2017).*

These ligaments are responsible to the restriction of these movements:

- **Iliotibial band**: this ligament serves as a ligamentous connection between the femur and the lateral tibia.
- **Anterior cruciate ligament**: Acts to limit the rotation and forward movement of the tibia.
- **Posterior cruciate ligament**: Acts to limit backward movement of the tibia.
- **Medial cruciate ligament**: Provides stability to the inner area of the knee.
- **Lateral cruciate ligament**: Provides stability to the outer area of the knee.

The round "donut-shaped" structures between the two big bones are the **meniscus**. They act as a shock absorber and distribute the weight that is transferred either during standing, walking or jumping. There is two menisci in each knee: the lateral meniscus and medial meniscus. Being able to absorb shock is crucial in protecting the knee and allows the femur and tibia to smoothly glide over each other.

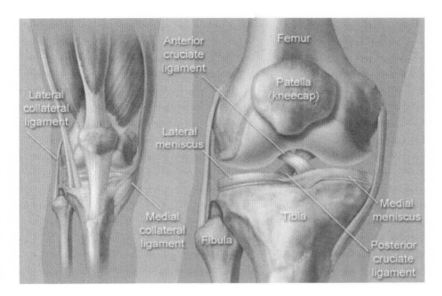

*Hoffman (2020).*

Understanding the kinetic chain of the knee joint

With rehabilitation of the knee we must consider the leg its relationship with the body as a whole. The knee is one of the most complicated structures in the body so caution is a must. For example, we must consider the other muscles and movement pattern during walking, running or even jumping. We must take into consideration of two factors:

1.) Above and below structures

Muscles surrounding the knee have a massive amount of influence on knee health and its rate of recovery. Muscles above the knee consist of hip flexors, quadriceps, hamstrings, internal and external hip rotators. Muscles below the knee consist of calf muscles, foot dorsiflexors, plantarflexors and muscles in the ankle and feet.

In the mid and later stages of knee rehabilitation, we incorporate multi-joint or compound movement into the program. Understanding the link between the knee and the rest of the body is important. As the body moves or bends in one direction, we must ask ourselves how does the knee translate? Is this movement pattern healthy or detrimental to the knee?

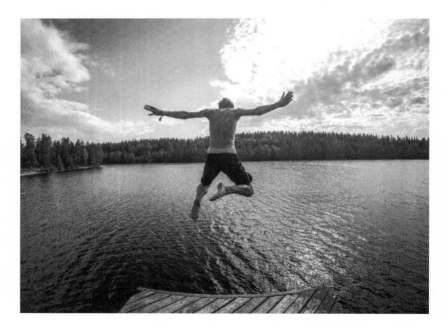

*Fornoni (2017).*

## 2.) Pronation of the knee

Understanding the relationship between the knee and the body is crucial because a collapse in one area will lead to a collapse in another area. For example pronation (rolling in) of the foot causes the knee to also roll inwards. This is known as knee **valgus**. This puts excessive pressure on the knee and will lead to motion compensations, friction, inflammation and eventually injury.

Thus, knee rehabilitation should also use a kinetic chain analysis to uncover any movement dysfunction. A dysfunctional movement pattern will still remain even after some pain at the knee has been alleviated. A corrective program at the end of specific rehabilitation will re-establish proper movement by having all related structures work together.

**If there is "shooting" pain down the back your leg, it might sciatica.**

Most often if you have lower back pain, you might have this "shooting" pain as well. It usually gets associated with one another injury but it's quite different. The reason why you feel this pain is because the nerve that runs from behind your hip down your leg is being compressed. This sensation can go to the buttocks, leg, calf or foot.

Often patients describe this pain as "shooting", an "electric shock" or "stabbing" pain. Of course each case is different but the general compression of the nerve remains the same.

Think of a garden hose with a slight fold in it. The water will still come out on the other end but not to its fullest potential. Like I always recommend if pain has subsided and is manageable – return to light exercise as soon as possible.

**Shins hurt? Could be shin splints.**

This is a very common exercise-related issue – mainly with sports with running and cutting. The term "shin-splints" refer to the pain around the big shin bone (tibia), more so on the inner edge.  It is the inflammation of muscles, tendon and bone tissues around the tibia where the muscles attach to the bone. Patients often report tenderness where the muscle connects to the bone.

Similar to many of the other injuries, it is caused by repetitive strain in the same area. Sports are the main cause of it; however, prolonged walking or running could cause it as well. Other causes of shin splints include having flat arches, high arches or wearing footwear with improper or poor support. Runners, dancers or athletes who jump a lot are at a higher risk of shin splints.

With acute care of this injury, use the classic P.R.I.C.E. protocol. This will bring down the pain and inflammation immediately. Secondly, look into getting orthotics and/or proper supporting footwear. Because running is very repetitive, it is a good idea to find something supportive and healthy for your feet to work in. Continuing to pound your feet and ankles in improper footwear can cause you to worsen your shin splints. Once some of the pain has subsided, see if you can return to exercise. You may still be feeling some soreness or discomfort in that area, but light movement and exercise will help. Getting the muscles, bones and tissues to function again is the best medicine you can give it.

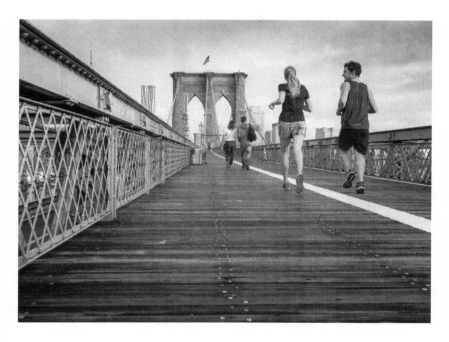

*MacNewton (2015).*

# Treatments

## Jumper's Knee (Patellar Tendonitis)

**Mobilize: Knee flexion presses:** *2 sets, 10 repetitions per side.*

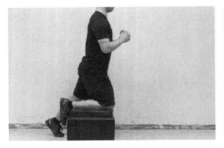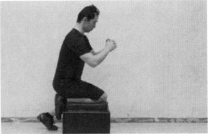

Pro-tip: This is a slow movement. Aim for 3 seconds down and 3 seconds up.

**Mobilize: Knee extension presses:** *2 sets, 10 repetitions.*

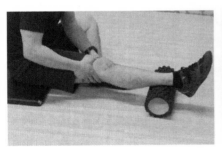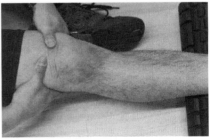

Pro-tip: You are gently pushing down on the thigh, right above the knee, trying to increase the range.

**Stabilize: Band hip flexion + extension:** *3 sets, 10 flexion + 10 extension per leg.*

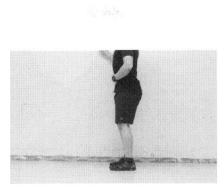
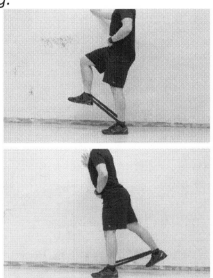

Pro-tip: Keep tall in the torso. You are working mainly hip muscles.

**Stabilize: Wall-sit:** *3 sets, 45 seconds.*

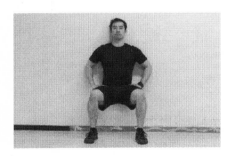

Pro-tip: Push the knees outwards. The weight of the body should be on the heels.

**Strengthen: Half squat holds:** *3 sets, 1 minute of hold.*

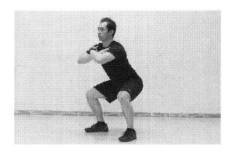

Pro-tip: You are stressing the quadriceps in this movement. Keep good posture.

**Strengthen: Raised heel squats:** *4 sets, 15 repetitions.*

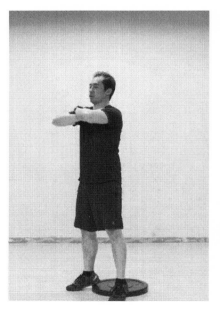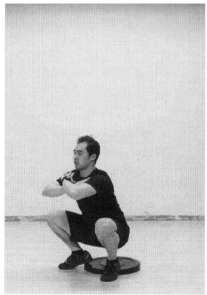

Pro-tip: Push the hips back as you squat down.

**Strengthen: Kneeling get-ups:** *4 sets, 10 repetitions per leg.*

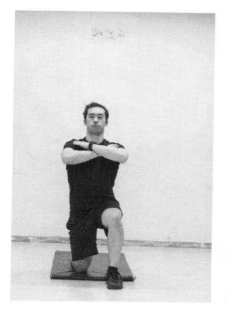 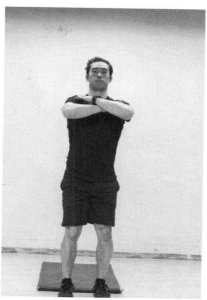

Pro-tip: Use the front leg to push off the ground, then stand tall.

**Strengthen: Seated leg extensions:** *4 sets, 20 repetitions.*

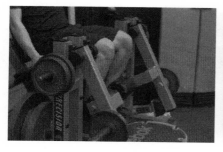 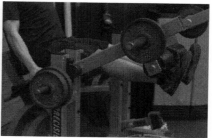

Pro-tip: Choose a lighter weight for this movement as you are targeting muscle endurance.

**Perpetuate: Dumbbell push-press:** *4 sets, 10 repetitions.*

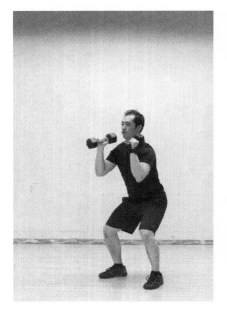 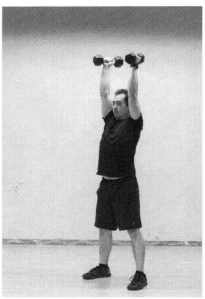

Pro-tip: Bend the knee only slightly before pushing off explosively, transferring the power into the arms and dumbbells.

**Perpetuate: Single-leg drop & hold:** *4 sets, 10 repetitions per leg.*

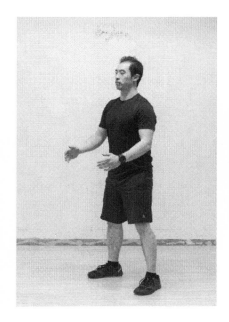 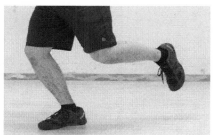

Pro-tip: Explosively drop the weight onto the targeted leg then catching it with a slight knee bend, absorbing the weight of the body.

**Perpetuate: Box jump:** *4 sets, 10 repetitions.*

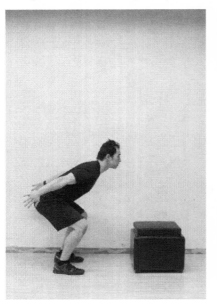 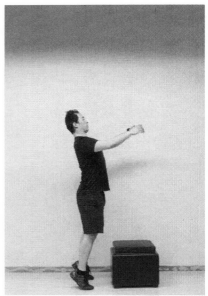

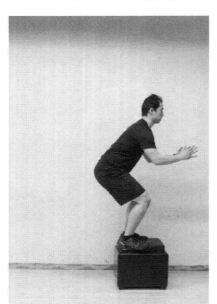

Pro-tip: Jump as naturally as possible. Land in an "athletic posture" - knees bent, chest out.

# Strained Hamstrings

**Mobilize: Active knee extensions:** *2 sets, 10 repetitions per side.*

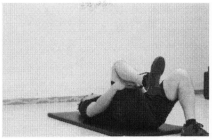 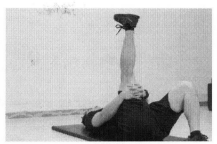

Pro-tip: Keep the upper leg frozen as you extend your lower leg.

**Mobilize: Band-assisted hamstrings stretch:** *2 sets, 10 repetitions per leg.*

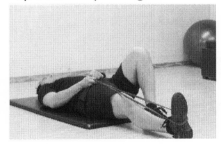 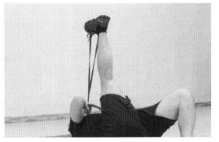

Pro-tip: Pull the leg up in a controlled speed. The band should help with the stretch.

**Stabilize: Split-stance holds:** *3 sets, 45 seconds of hold per side.*

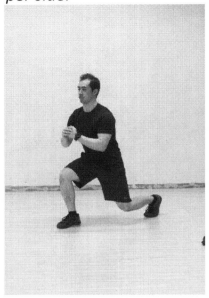

Pro-tip: Keep the torso upright and bend the back leg.

**Stabilize: Prone bent-leg extensions:** *3 sets, 10 repetitions per side.*

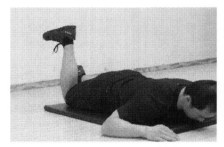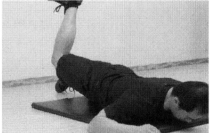

Pro-tip: Try to keep the hips flat on the ground. You are engaging your glutes.

**Stabilize: Glute bridge marches:** *3 sets, 10 repetitions per leg.*

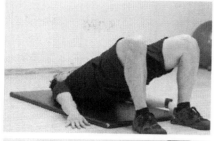 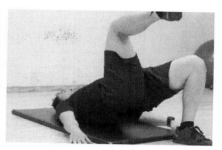

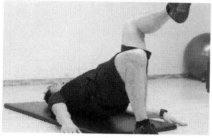

Pro-tip: Start with the glute bridge then keep the hips up as you alternate lifting legs.

**Strengthen: Frog pumps:** *4 sets, 15 repetitions.*

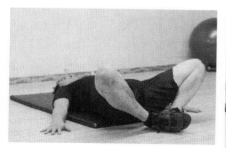 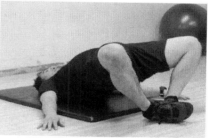

Pro-tip: Push at the heels and clench the butt-cheeks at the top.

**Strengthen: Single-leg Romanian hinges:** *4 sets, 10 repetitions per leg.*

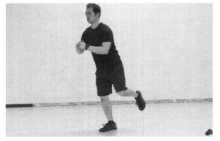 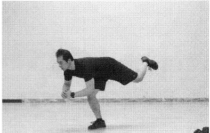

Pro-tip: Keep a slight bend in the supporting leg and bend at the waist.

**Strengthen: Hyperextensions:** *4 sets, 10 repetitions.*

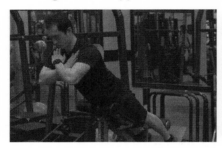 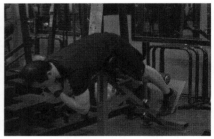

Pro-tip: Squeeze the butt-cheeks as you lift the torso up. Add weight for progression.

**Strengthen: Swiss ball hamstring curls:** *4 sets, 10 repetitions.*

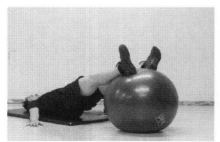 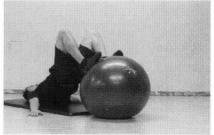

Pro-tip: Keep the hips lifted during the entire set.

**Perpetuate: Dumbbell reverse lunges:** *4 sets, 10 repetitions per leg.*

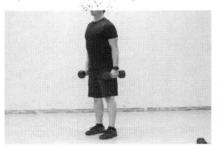 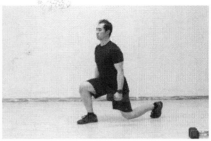

Pro-tip: Keep the body upright and bend the back leg. You can choose a heavier weight for this movement.

**Perpetuate: Dumbbell Romanian deadlifts:** *4 sets, 15 repetitions.*

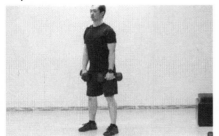 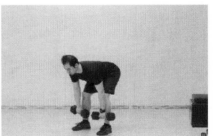

Pro-tip: Push the hips back, get a slight bend in the knee and keep the back straight.

**Perpetuate: Rocket jump + absorb:** *4 sets, 5 repetitions.*

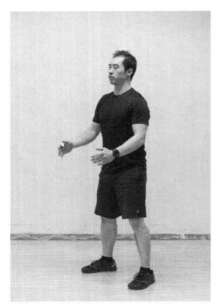 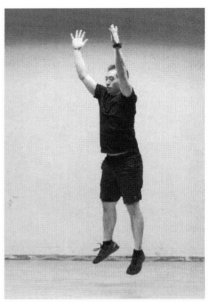

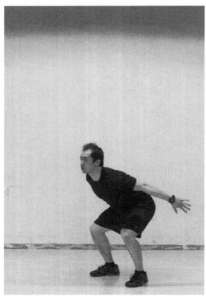

Pro-tip: Always land in an "athletic posture" - knees bent and pushed out; slight forward lean.

# Torn Meniscus

**Mobilize: Meniscus glide:** *2 sets, 5 repetitions per side.*

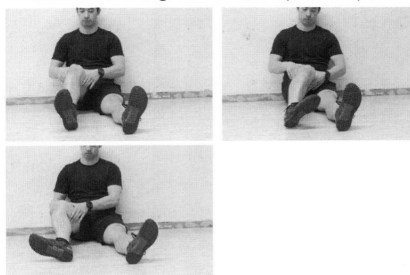

Pro-tip: You are rotating at the feet and lower leg. Your upper leg is frozen.

**Stabilize: Wall sit:** *3 sets, 45 seconds.*

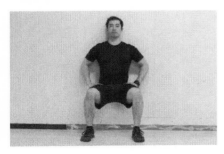

Pro-tip: Drive the knees outwards and keep still. Go as far as pain will allow it.

**Stabilize: Single-leg balance:** *2 sets, 30 seconds each leg.*

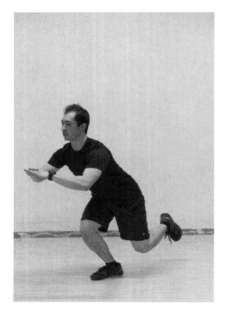

Pro-tip: Only a 25% bend is needed. Lean forward with the body.

**Stabilize: Bosu-ball balance:** *2 sets, 30 seconds per leg.*

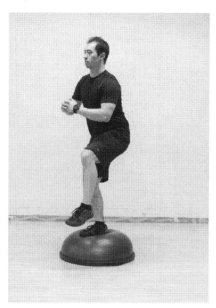

Pro-tip: Slight bend of the standing knee is required.

**Strengthen: Glute bridge with dorsiflexion + plantarflexion:** *4 sets, 20 repetitions each.*

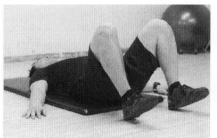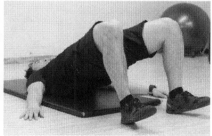

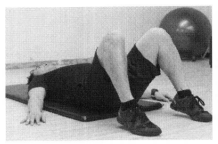 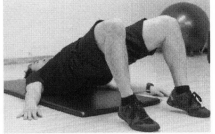

Pro-tip: The knees should always be pushed outwards.

## Strengthen: Glute bridge with torso roll: *4 sets, 5 repetitions per side.*

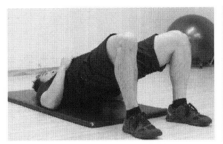 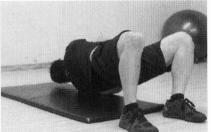

Pro-tip: Begin with the glute bridge then reach with the hand to the opposite side. Keep the legs still. Keep the hips up while reaching.

## Strengthen: Band resisted single-leg hip-hinges: *4 sets, 10 repetitions per side.*

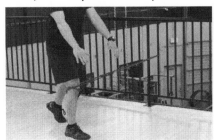 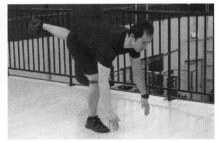

Pro-tip: Slight bend of the knee is needed. Keep the back straight. Keep the knee stacked on top of the ankle.

**Perpetuate: Goblet squat with hold at bottom:** *4 sets, 15 repetitions.*

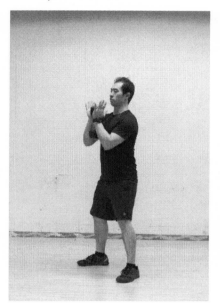 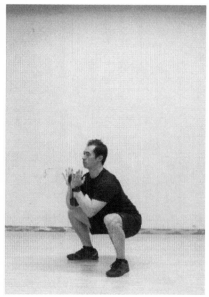

Pro-tip: You can choose a slightly heavier weight for this. Aim to hold for 2 full seconds at the bottom of the squat.

**Perpetuate: Single-leg quarter squats:** *4 sets, 10 repetitions per leg.*

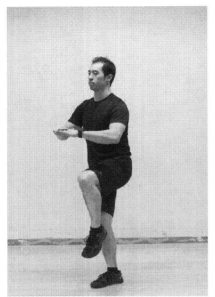 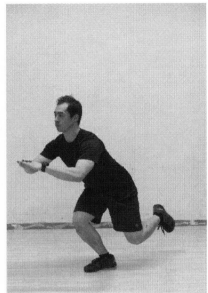

Pro-tip: Push the hips back as you bend the knee. Add weight for progression. Go slowly.

**Perpetuate: Jogging in place:** *4 sets, 45 seconds of jogging.*

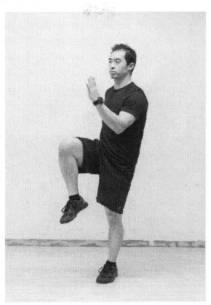

Pro-tip: Keep a tall posture during the movement. Be mindful of the knee position and ground impact.

## Torn ACL or PCL

**Mobilize: Band assisted heel slides:** *2 sets, 10 repetitions per side.*

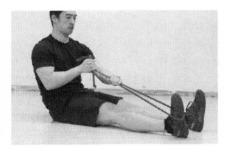 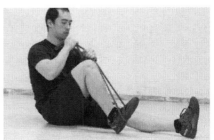

Pro-tip: You are working both hamstrings and quads in this movement.

## Mobilize: Foam roll quads, hamstrings + calves: *2 sets, 30 seconds per area.*

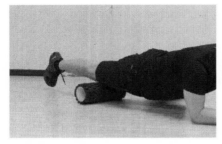
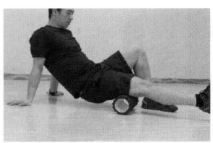
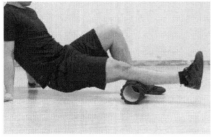

Pro-tip: Keep rolling until you find a tender area then stay on it until it goes down.

## Stabilize: Lying straight-leg raise: *3 sets, 10 repetitions.*

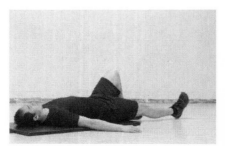
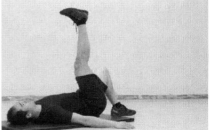

Pro-tip: Raise and lower the leg in a controller manner; aim for 3 seconds up and 3 seconds down.

### Stabilize: Single-leg balance and hold with band: *3 sets, 30 seconds hold.*

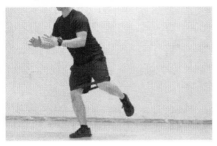

Pro-tip: The band goes an inch above the knee caps. A slight bend in the knee is needed.

### Stabilize: Rear-leg elevated hinges: *3 sets, 10 repetitions per leg.*

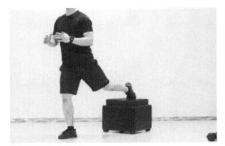 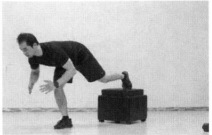

Pro-tip: Slight bend in both legs are needed. Keep the back straight and bend at the hips.

### Strengthen: Box heel taps: *4 sets, 10 repetitions per leg.*

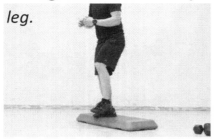 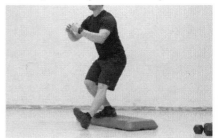

Pro-tip: Keep a tall posture. Lightly tap the heel under controlled.

### Strengthen: Swiss ball hamstring curls: *4 sets, 15 repetitions.*

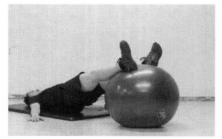 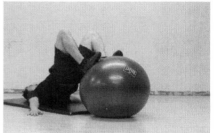

Pro-tip: Keep the hips up and the glutes squeezed during the set.

### Strengthen: Single-leg glute bridges: *4 sets, 10 repetitions per leg.*

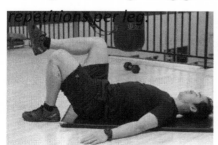 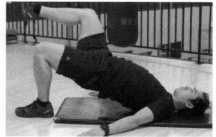

Pro-tip: Drive the heels into the ground as you left the hips up.

**Strengthen: Trap-bar deadlifts:** *4 sets, 10 repetitions.*

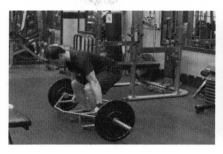 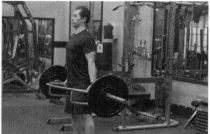

Pro-tip: You can choose a heavier weight to challenge the lower body.

**Perpetuate: Box pistol squat:** *4 sets, 10 repetitions per side.*

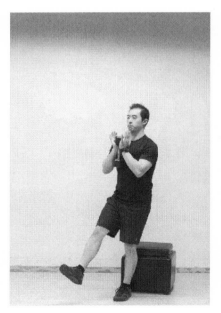 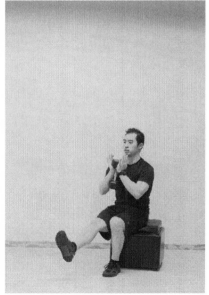

Pro-tip: Choose a lighter weight for this movement. You can adjust the height of the box depending on the progression and height of the person.

## Perpetuate: Single-leg jump + absorb: *4 sets, 5 repetitions per leg.*

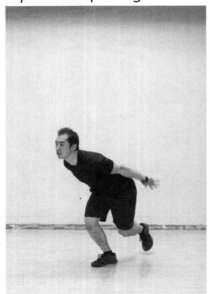 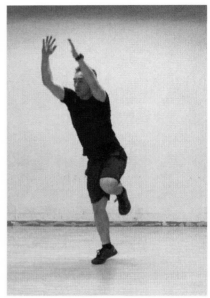

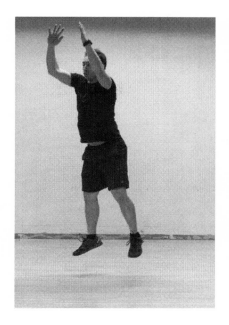 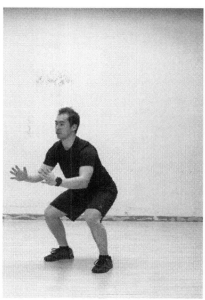

Pro-tip: Take off with one leg but land with two in an athletic stance.

**Perpetuate: Skater jumps:** *4 sets, 5 repetition per leg.*

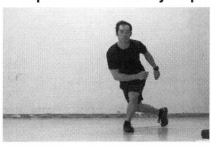 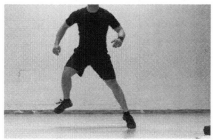

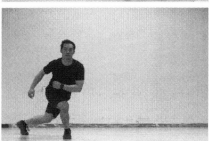

Pro-tip: Push off explosively and land in a controlled fashion. Be mindful of knee position and landing impact.

# Shin-Splints

## Mobilize: Dynamic Japanese-sit stretch: *2 sets, 10 repetitions.*

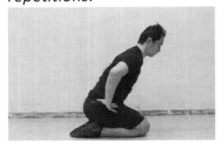 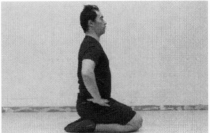

Pro-tip: Keep the top of the foot in contact with the floor throughout the movement.

## Mobilize: Foam roll tibialis anterior and calf: *2 sets, 30 seconds per area.*

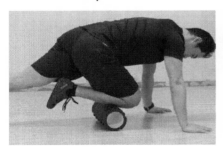 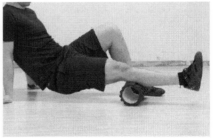

Pro-tip: Roll until you find a tender area then keep the pressure on it.

**Stabilize: Open-chain heel circles:** *3 sets, 10 repetition per direction.*

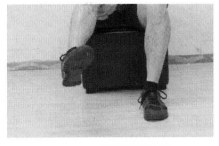
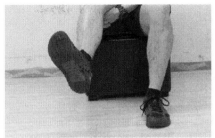
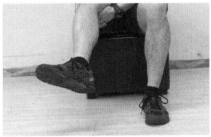

Pro-tip: You are making circles leading with the heel.

**Strengthen: Heel walks:** *3 sets, 45 seconds of walk.*

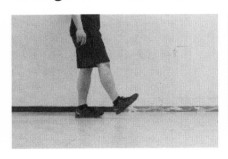
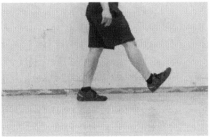

Pro-tip: Keep the toes peeled up as high as possible throughout the entire set.

## Strengthen: Toe walks: *3 sets, 45 seconds of walk.*

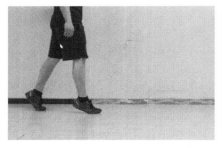 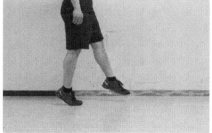

Pro-tip: Keep the ankle flexed as high as possible throughout the entire set.

## Strengthen: Calf raises: *4 sets, 20 repetitions.*

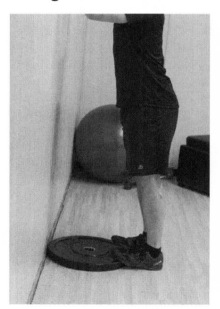 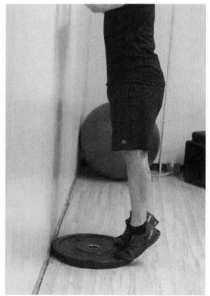

Pro-tip: The heels must touch the floor between each repetition.

**Perpetuate: Rapid calf jumps:** *4 sets, 20 repetitions.*

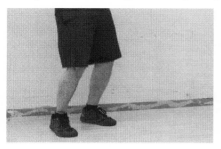 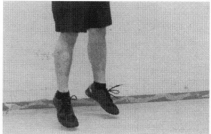

Pro-tip: Bend the knee at a minimum. Most of the movement happens at the ankles.

**Perpetuate: Forward bound with hold:** *4 sets, 5 repetitions per leg.*

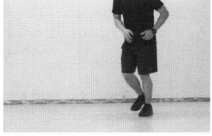 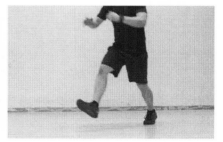

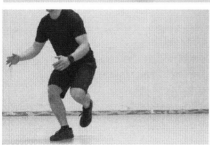

Pro-tip: Absorb the landing in a controlled way keeping high tension in the ankle.

**Perpetuate: Skater jumps:** *4 sets, 5 repetitions per side.*

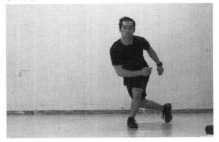 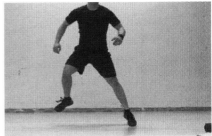

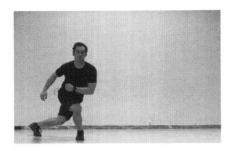

Pro-tip: Control the landing and keep tension in the ankles.

## Staple Stretches

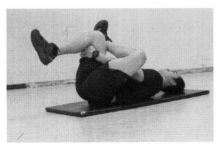 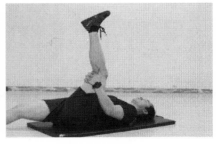

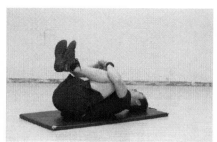 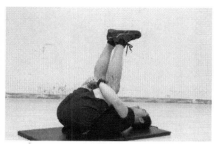

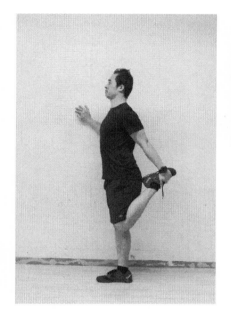 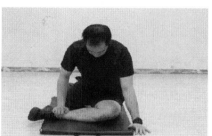

# **9.** Ankle and feet injuries

## Ankle Science

Like the knee, the ankle is another complex mechanism that aids us in everyday tasks. The ankle is actually composed of two joints: the true ankle joint and the subtalar joint. The true ankle joint is made of three bones: the tibia, fibula and the talus. The true joint is responsible of the up-and-down of the ankle.

Beneath the true ankle joint is the subtalar joint. This joint is made of the talus on top and the calcaneus on the bottom. This joint allows side-to-side movement of the foot. Ends of these bones are covered by articular cartilage that provides smooth movements.

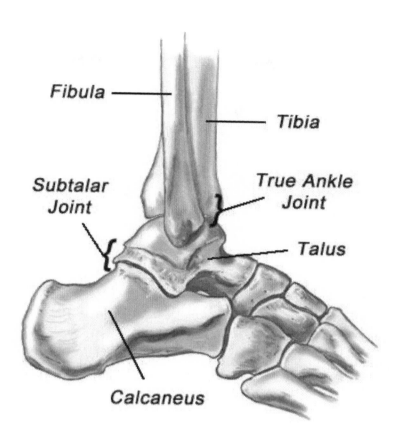

Fibula

Tibia

Subtalar Joint

True Ankle Joint

Talus

Calcaneus

*Kidport (2012).*

There are numerous of ligaments that connect the different bones in the foot. One ligament that is worth noting is the anterior talofibular ligament. This is the first and/or only ligament to be injured in the majority of ankle sprains. It also has the highest risk of injury during an ankle sprain.

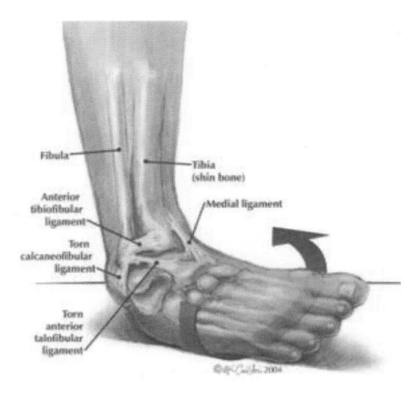

*Racich (2015).*

<u>UN-sprain these ligaments</u>

Now we are getting a little more in-depth with sprained ankle ligaments. A "sprained ankle" is when the supporting structures (the ligaments) are pushed beyond their limits and tear. Most mild sprains can be treated initial with the P.R.I.C.E. protocol. However, the rehabilitation portion is a whole different ball game.

Most of the ankle sprains people experience is the lateral ankle sprain – possible 90% of sprains are this time. Although rare, some people have sprained medial tendons. As mentioned above, one of the most sprained ligament is the anterior talofibular ligament – along with the posterior talofibular ligament and the calcaneofibular ligament. Regardless which tendon we sprain or how fancy their names sound, we must focus on the rehabilitation process in order to regain full range-of-motion and strength.

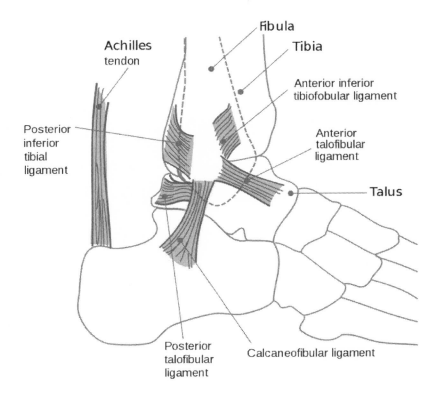

*Wikipedia (2020).*

Biggest tendon in the body?

The Achilles tendon – the strongest and largest tendon in the body. It is also known as a co-jointed tendon; it is jointed directly into the calf muscles. The Achilles tendon is a key player because its job is to transmit force into the ankle and feet generated by the calf muscles.

The Achilles tendon is very dense and is under constant tension. Because of this reason, this area has the poorest blood supply making it susceptible to injury and incredibly slow to heal after injury.

Common injuries to the Achilles tendon:

- Achilles tendonitis
  - This refers to the presence of inflammation in the Achilles. Often patients will report tenderness, pain and swelling in the area right above the heel. Most often caused by wearing high heels, running up hills, jumping or activities that require a sudden burst of speed.
- Tendinosis
  - This is simply degeneration in the Achilles Tendon due to a previous tear. You can diagnose this by feeling a "tendon nodule" very close to the heel. This nodule is formed by the accumulation of scar tissue from the last tear.
- Rupture of the tendon – partial or complete
  - This is ripping or separation of the tendon at the calcaneus (heel bone). The Achilles Tendon is able to withstand a force of a thousand pounds without tearing, however, it is the second most frequently ruptured tendon in the body.

At the Achilles Tendon, or any tendon for that matter, there is often a poor oxygen supply due to low levels of blood vessels. This causes a low traffic of delivery of nutrients and removal of wastes. This ultimately results in poor healing and the thickening of the tendon. Chronic tendinosis can lead to a complete rupture of the tendon if not properly treated and taken care of.

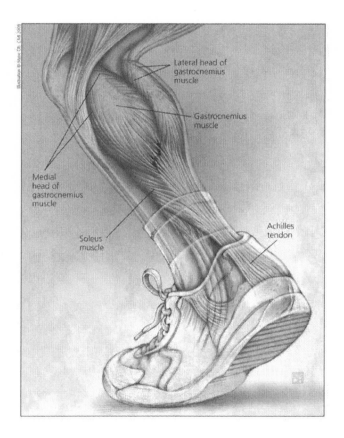

*Krych (2011).*

<u>Run a lot? Got burning in the feet?</u>

Then you probably have a case of plantar fasciitis. You may also have one or more of the following symptoms:

- Heel pain in the first few steps in the morning.
- Dull aching or sharp pain in the heel.
- A pulling sensation in the hell up into the Achilles.

Usually individuals who get plantar fasciitis are runners, football players and workers who stand and/or walk for prolong periods of time. With long working hours, a high amount of stress go into the feet and supporting structures. Plantar fasciitis can also be caused by flat or excessively high arches, being overweight, weak foot muscles or poor/mis-fitted shoes.

What is it exactly? It is simply the inflammation (suffix "itis") of the plantar fascia. This fascia is a thin band that runs from the heel bone to the toes. It is also the deeper soft-tissues structures that show signs of injury so you would want to protect this structure. Plantar fasciitis typically develops over a long period of time through prolonged stress and abuse of the feet.

A few notable causes of this inflammation are the following:

- Muscle imbalances in the body.
- Abnormal foot biomechanics.
- Repetitive strain motions in the lower body.
- Inadequate support in the shoe and/or aches.
- Acute trauma to the feet.

As mentioned above, majority of these causes are repeated stresses so as a result, this fascia and surrounding tissues can develop micro-tears. If you do not get the proper amount of rest, they can become inflamed and damaged. When they become inflamed, the body lays down scar tissues in order to facilitate healing which results in the shortening of the plantar flexors. Further complications can include calf and hamstring muscle restrictions as well as problems with the internal and external rotators of the hip.

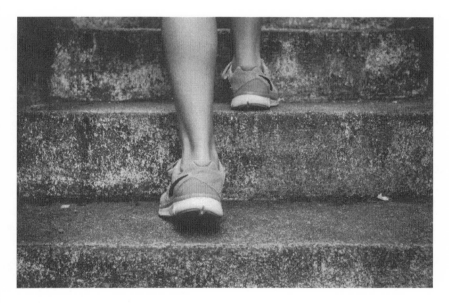

*Nascimento (2016).*

# Treatments

## Ankle Sprain

**Mobilize: Open-chain heel circles:** *2 sets, 10 repetitions per direction.*

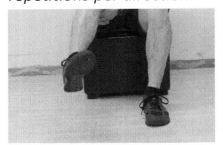
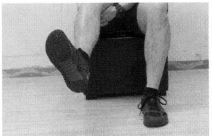

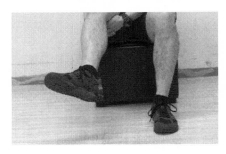

Pro-tip: You are making circles leading with the heel. Maximum range-of-motion as possible.

**Mobilize: Wall dorsiflexion press:** *2 sets, 10 repetitions per leg.*

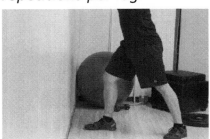
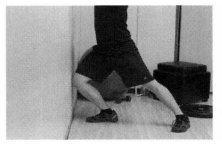

Pro-tip: Keep the heel planted on the floor at all times.

## Mobilize: Squat body shifts: *2 sets, 5 repetitions per side.*

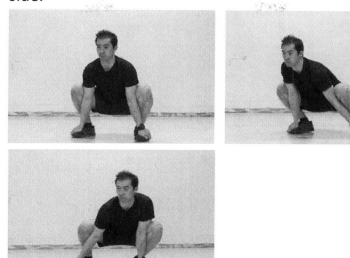

Pro-tip: You are rocking your body left and right, trying to increase the range-of-motion to the sides.

**Stabilize: Bosu-ball balances:** *3 sets, 45 seconds of balance.*

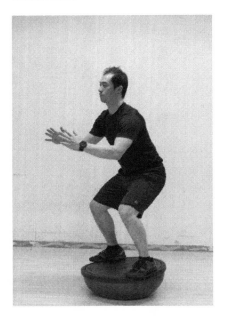

Pro-tip: Keep the tension on the ankles.

**Stabilize: Rear leg elevated hip-hinges:** *3 sets, 10 repetitions per side.*

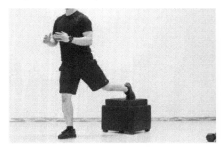 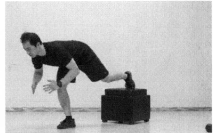

Pro-tip: Keep a slight bend in the knee and keep tension in the ankle.

**Strengthen: Single-leg Romanian deadlifts:** *4 sets, 10 repetitions per side.*

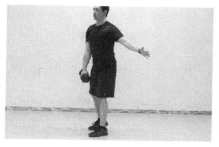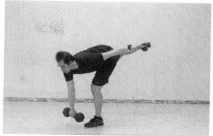

Pro-tip: You are challenging the balance in the ankle. Keep a slight bend in the knee.

**Strengthen: Step-ups:** *4 sets, 10 repetitions per side.*

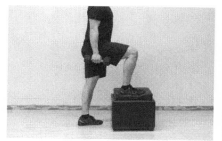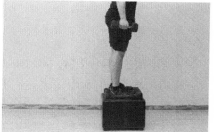

Pro-tip: Add more weight for progression. Keep the ankles stiff during the step.

**Strengthen: Smite machine calf eccentrics:** *4 sets, 15 repetitions.*

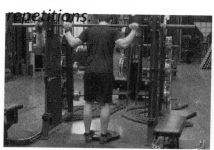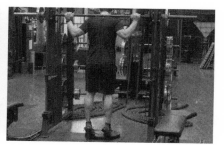

Pro-tip: Aim for a 3 second lowering phase. The heel must touch the floor between reps.

## Strengthen: Single calf raises: *4 sets, 15 repetitions per leg.*

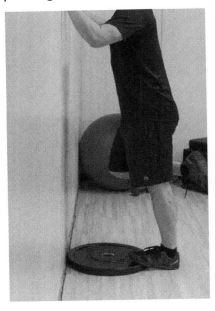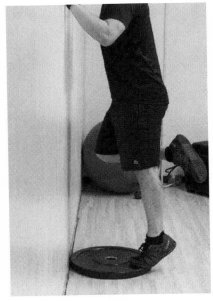

Pro-tip: Move through a controlled pace. The heel must touch the floor between reps.

## Perpetuate: Forward lunges: *4 sets, 10 repetitions per leg.*

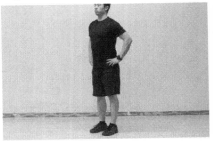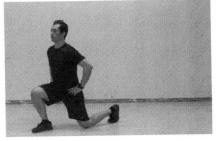

Pro-tip: Keep the body upright when lunging. Keep tension in the ankle during the step. Add weight for progression

**Perpetuate: Marches:** *4 sets, 45 seconds.*

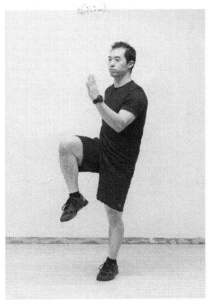

Pro-tip: Keep the tension in the ankle with each step. Progress to running on the spot.

**Perpetuate: Bound and hold:** *4 sets, 5 repetitions per leg.*

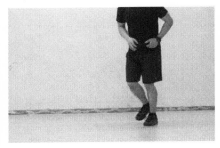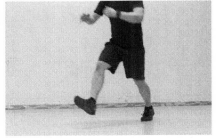

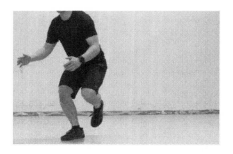

Pro-tip: Absorb the landing in a controlled manner.

# Achilles Tendon Rupture

**Mobilize: Foam roll calves:** *2 sets, 45 seconds per leg.*

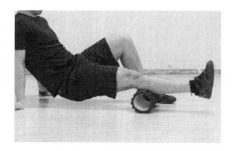

Pro-tip: Roll until you find a tender spot then stay on it until the stiffness goes away.

**Mobilize: Lacrosse ball smash arch of foot:** *2 sets, 30 seconds each leg.*

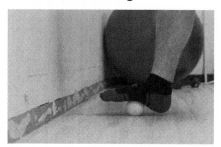

Pro-tip: Roll until you find a tender spot then stay on it until the stiffness goes away.

**Mobilize: Dynamic wall calf stretch:** *2 sets, 10 repetitions per leg.*

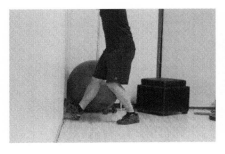 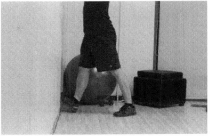

Pro-tip: Move in a smooth and controlled pace; keep it moving and fluid (non-stop).

**Stabilize: Alternating single leg balance:** *2 sets, 10 per leg.*

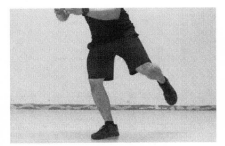 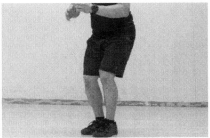

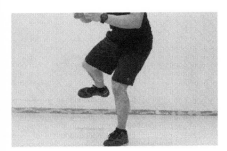

Pro-tip: Aim for a 3 second hold per leg; you are challenging the ankles ability to balance.

**Stabilize: Bosu-ball balance:** *2 sets, 45 seconds of hold.*

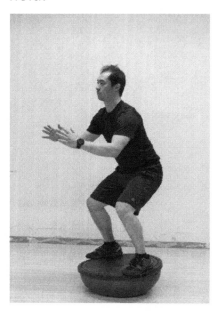

Pro-tip: Push the knees out. You are challenging the muscles in the foot.

**Strengthen: Single-leg deadlift:** *4 sets, 10 repetitions per leg.*

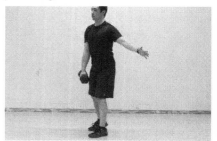 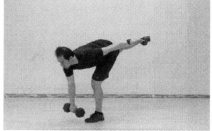

Pro-tip: Keep a slight bend in the standing leg.

## Strengthen: Toe-off walks: *4 sets, 45 seconds.*

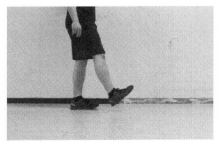 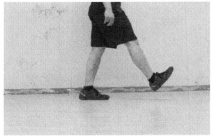

Pro-tip: Peel the toes up as high as you can for both legs.

## Strengthen: Raised heel calf raises: *4 sets, 20 repetitions.*

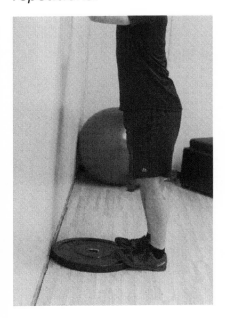 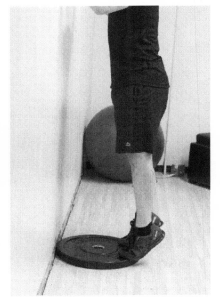

Pro-tip: Stand tall and the heels must touch the floor between every repetition.

**Strengthen: Stair climb:** *4 sets, 45 seconds of climb.*

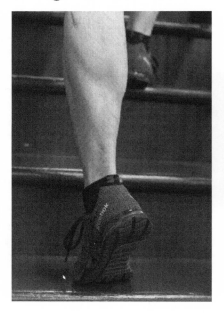 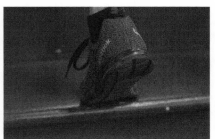

Pro-tip: Focus on the toe-off phase of the step.

**Perpetuate: Goblet squats:** *4 sets, 15 repetitions.*

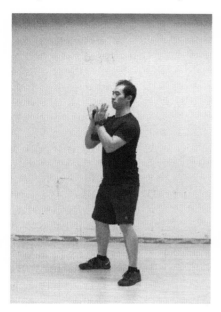 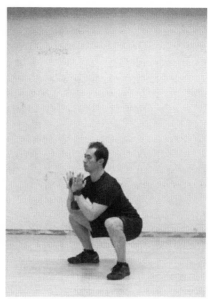

Pro-tip: You can choose a heavier weight for this movement.

**Perpetuate: Step ups:** *4 sets, 10 repetitions per leg.*

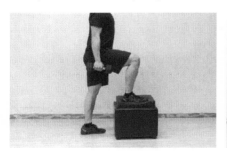 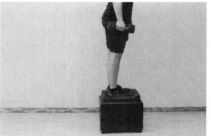

Pro-tip: You can choose a heavier weight for this movement.

**Perpetuate: Single-leg jump and absorb:** *4 sets, 5 repetitions per leg.*

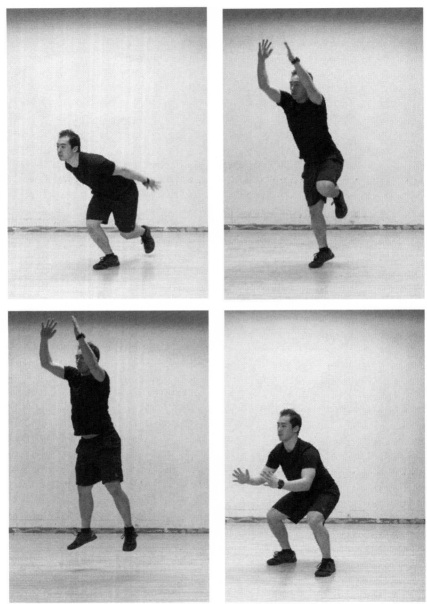

Pro-tip: Land in an athletic stance; knees bend and chest out.

# Plantar Fasciitis

**Mobilize: Lacrosse ball smash on heel:** *2 sets, 45 seconds per foot.*

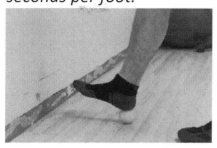

Pro-tip: You are loosening the fibers in the heel.

**Stabilize: Big toe flexion ankle plantarflexion + heel raise:** *2 sets, 10 reps of each.*

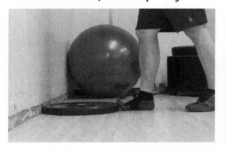
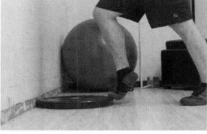
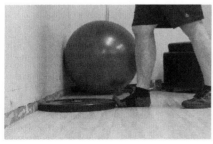
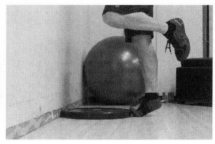

Pro-tip: Keep the toes flexed on the plate as you move at the ankle.

**Strengthen: Arch strengthening:** *3 sets, 30 seconds of hold.*

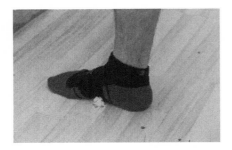

Pro-tip: You are lifting the arch so that the ball of paper fits underneath.

**Strengthen: Heel drops + calf raises:** *4 sets, 20 reps of each movement.*

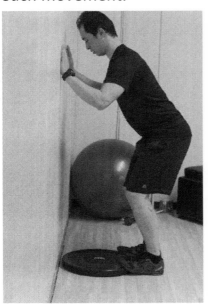
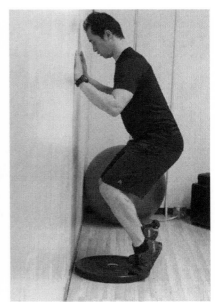

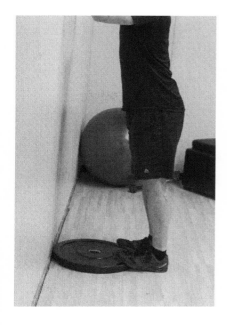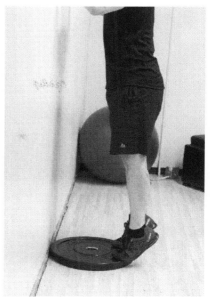

Pro-tip: Do 20 of knees bent then 20 with knees straight - that is 1 set.

## Perpetuate: Lateral lunges: *4 sets, 10 repetitions per side.*

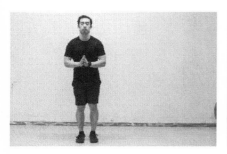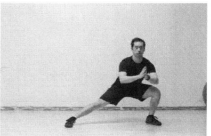

Pro-tip: Push the knee out and the hips back.

**Perpetuate: Forward drop and absorb:** *4 sets, 5 repetitions.*

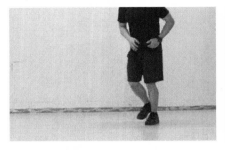 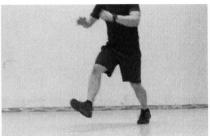

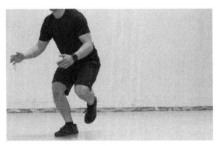

Pro-tip: Keep the foot and toes stiff upon landing.

**Perpetuate: Skip on the spot:** *4 sets, 30 seconds of skipping.*

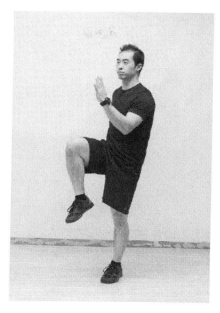

Pro-tip: Keep the movement athletic and natural.

## High Ankle Sprain

**Mobilize: Banded joint distraction:** *2 sets, 10 repetitions.*

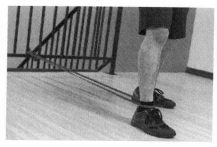 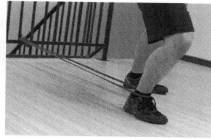

Pro-tip: Allow the band to pull the ankle joint back while the knee goes forward.

## Mobilize: "Sad man" squats: *2 sets, 10 repetitions.*

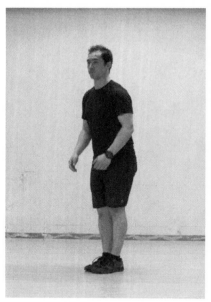
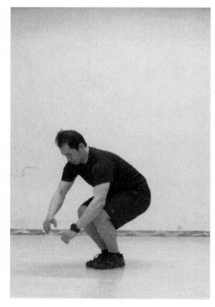
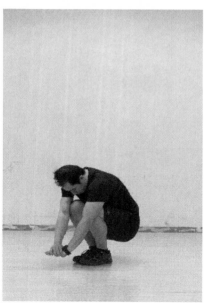

Pro-tip: Keep the heels on the floor and keep the movement fluid and dynamic.

### Stabilize: Tandem walking: *3 sets, 45 seconds.*

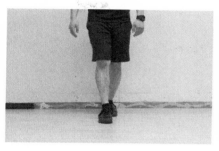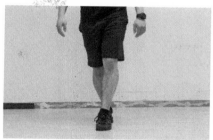

Pro-tip: Walking in a straight line with the heel touching the toes each step.

### Stabilize: Banded hip abduction balances: *3 sets, 45 seconds.*

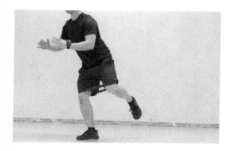

Pro-tip: Keep a slight bend in the standing leg.

**Strengthen: Heel walks:** *4 sets, 45 seconds.*

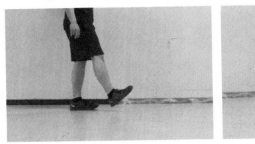 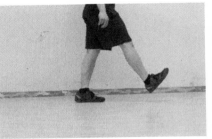

Pro-tip: Keep the toes on both legs pulled up at all times.

**Strengthen: Monster Walks:** *4 sets, 10 repetitions.*

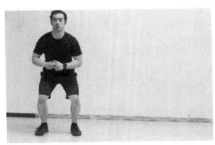 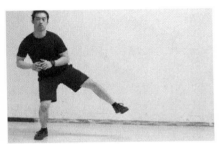

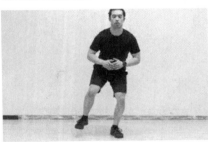

Pro-tip: Work on loading the ankles slowly and gradually.

**Strengthen: Goblet squats:** *4 sets, 15 repetitions.*

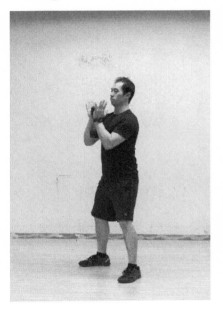 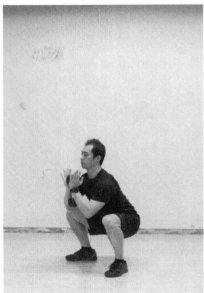

Pro-tip: Drive the knees out and push the hips back.

**Strengthen: Calf raises on Smith machine:** *4 sets, 15 repetitions.*

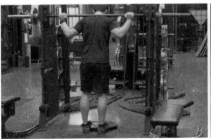 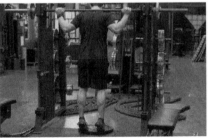

Pro-tip: The heels must touch the floor between every rep.

**Perpetuate: Lateral lunge shifts:** *4 sets, 10 repetitions.*

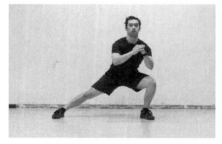 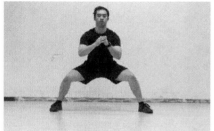

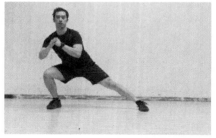

Pro-tip: Push the knees out. Add weight for progression.

**Perpetuate: Single-leg Romanian deadlift:** *4 sets, 10 repetitions per leg.*

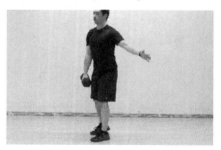 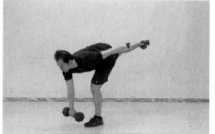

Pro-tip: Keep a slight bend in the standing leg.

**Perpetuate: Rocket Jump:** *4 sets, 5 repetitions.*

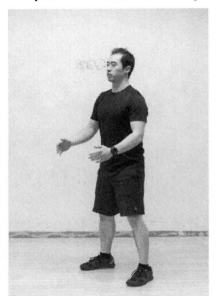
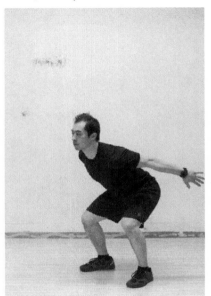
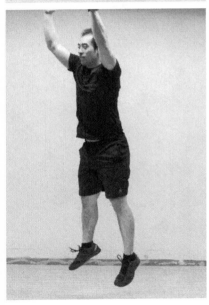

Pro-tip: Jump up explosively and land in an athletic position; absorbing the impact.

# Staple Stretches

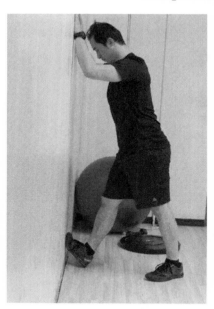
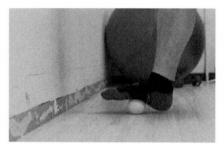
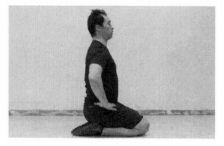

# **10.** What is Next? The Ultimate Progression

You have successfully recovered from your injury. The pain has subsided and you have regained most of your mobility and range-of-motion. The instability in that joint is no longer an issue and you have recovered most of your functional strength. So now what? What is the next step?

You must MAINTAIN it. In my experience treating patients, most patients stop making progress (or even regress) because they fail to keep up with their program. I am giving you these tools for you to use as often as you can. The more you utilize these tools the longer you will stay pain-free and perhaps get even stronger. The LESS you keep up with your program, the higher chances of a relapse.

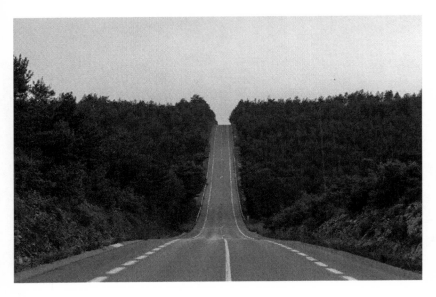

*Aldyrkhanov (2018).*

And why would you want to relapse? You worked so hard to make the progress; keep working at it to make it stick. The key-word here is LONGEVITY. Think life-long with the progress. A three or six month program will not cut it. Get used to a program that lasts a year or two. Be relapse free and train for the long-term.

We have fixed your wings and now you are free to fly wherever you wish. This is where you can branch out after an injury setback. Options are endless here. Some may decide they want to return to yoga. Some may want to start a career in powerlifting. Some may resume a spin class after a knee injury. Whatever you choose, you can head in that direction with the tools and knowledge you have gained. The ULTIMATE PROGRESSION is to return to the activities you love and to do them with no fear of re-injury.

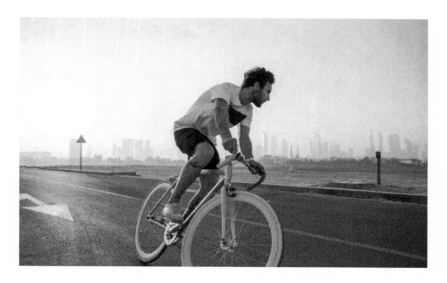

*Kennaugh (2018).*

With future activities it is critical that you be mindful of your past injury history. When you have injured an area, unfortunately, it will never be the same again. This is because rehabilitation and healing brings along complications. One of those complications are the laying of scar tissue. This can severely restrict mobility which may lead to compensation with the opposing limb, which will lead to an imbalance in the body and may ultimately lead to a RE-injury. The take-away point is to be mindful of past injuries as you embark on any future physical activities.

I hope this book has given you the tools needed to fix your injury. Remember that longevity of optimal health and performance is priority. Train hard to be PAIN-FREE, STRONG and YOUNG FOREVER.

Until next time,

# Coach Marco
Bachelor of Kinesiology
NSCA - Certified Personal Trainer

# About the Author

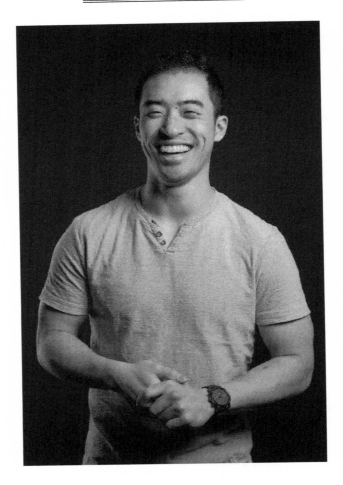

Coach Marco resides in British Columbia, Canada servicing the people around the Lower Mainland. His passion for movement and rehabilitation stems from his young roots practicing martial arts. From there he expanded into other recreational sports such as ice hockey, dodgeball and ultimate Frisbee.

He attended the University of British Columbia to obtain his Bachelors of Kinesiology; focusing on subjects such as biomechanics, anatomy and exercise physiology. Post-graduation, he worked in the field of personal training where he is able to apply his knowledge of exercise science.

Today he works as a registered kinesiologist, serving patients across the Vancouver city and furthering his experience in human movement and rehabilitation. Coach Marco has been in the field of rehab for four years and have been in the field of fitness for seven years. He's always looking to hone his craft and to practice with even more depth.

# References

Mahapatra, Anupam (2019). Unsplash. *Photos for everyone.*
https://unsplash.com/photos/Vz0RbclzG_w

Form (2019). Unsplash. *Photos for everyone.*
https://unsplash.com/photos/w0YIvob3LlI

Matt Jones (2015) on Unsplash. *Photos for everyone.*
https://unsplash.com/photos/N6szxrwGOOo

Alex Kotliarsky (2017). Unsplash. *Photos for everyone.*
https://unsplash.com/photos/ourQHRTE2IM

Mirko Blicke (2017). Unsplash. *Photos for everyone.*
https://unsplash.com/photos/V_y81v_lI4k

Vicky Sim (2017). Unsplash. *Photos for everyone.*
https://unsplash.com/photos/gxOIwb9vzIc

Zac Durant (2017). Unsplash. *Photos for everyone.*
https://unsplash.com/photos/_6HzPU9Hyfg

Zoltan Tasi (2017). Unsplash. *Photos for everyone.*
https://unsplash.com/photos/EpTbPG9yQg0

Upper cervical chiropractic of Monmouth (2019). *Upper cervical chiropractic of Monmouth.* Retrieved from
https://getwellnj.com/top-5-neck-pain-prevention-tips/

Adelaide West Physiotherapy and Pilates Classes (2018). *Adelaide West Physiotherapy and Pilates Classes.* Retrieved from https://phyxphysio.com.au/blog/reasons-keep-good-posture/

David Jockers (2014). *Live well chiropractic*. Retrieved from https://livewellchiro.com.au/bad-posture-equals-bad-health/

Alpha Spine Center (2019). *Alpha Spine Center*. Retrieved from https://www.alphaspinecenter.com/newsletter-blog/upper-lower-cross-syndrome

pt Health (2018). *pt Health*. Retrieved from https://www.pthealth.ca/conditions/whiplash/

Chuttersnap (2018). Unsplash. *Photos for everyone*. https://unsplash.com/photos/rsEiUMyvtuo

Pamela Thompson (2019). *Vallarata Tribune*. Retrieved from https://vallartatribune.com/shoulder-pain/

Jeff Williams (2019). *Jeff Williams PT*. Retrieved from https://www.jeffwilliamspt.com/2019/01/best-rotator-cuff-strengthening.html

The shoulder clinic of Idaho (2020). *The shoulder clinic of Idaho*. Retrieved from https://www.shoulderclinicofidaho.com/ac-joint-injuries-and-shoulder-separations/

Mayo Clinic Staff (2020). *Mayo Clinic*. Retrieved from https://www.mayoclinic.org/diseases-conditions/dislocated-shoulder/symptoms-causes/syc-20371715

Form (2017). Unsplashed. *Photos for everyone*. Retrieved from https://unsplash.com/photos/QP84K2HuIMY

Girish Khera (2016). Scientific Animations. *We make you look good*. Retrieved from
https://www.scientificanimations.com/setbacktocomeback-tennis-elbow-golfers-elbow-primer/

Orthoinfo (2020). Orthoinfo. *Carpal Tunnel Syndrome*. Retrieved from https://orthoinfo.aaos.org/en/diseases--conditions/carpal-tunnel-syndrome/

Noble, Ian (2019). Unsplash. *Photos for everyone*. Retrieved from https://unsplash.com/photos/pVrIREXWvks

eMedicineHealth (2019). eMedicineHealth. *Low Back Pain*. Retrieved from
https://www.emedicinehealth.com/back_pain_health/article_em.htm

Physio-pedia (2020). Physio-pedia. *Lower Crossed Syndrome*. Retrieved from https://www.physio-pedia.com/Lower_Crossed_Syndrome

Sastre, Erica (2019). Norwalk Sport & Spine. *Q: What is my Piriformis Muscle?* Retrieved from
https://www.norwalksportsandspine.com/qanda/category/exercise

Hills, Jake (2014). Unsplash. *Photos for everyone*. Retrieved from https://unsplash.com/photos/bt-Sc22W-BE

Westcoast SCI (2018). *Westcoast SCI*. Retrieved from https://westcoastsci.com/general-blog/2018/4/12/what-is-foam-rolling-and-how-to-use-one

Grauer, Yael (2016). Experience Life. *Expert Answers: Safe Rotational Exercises:* https://experiencelife.com/article/expert-answers-safe-rotational-exercises/

Calderone, Erin (2019). Oxygen. *4 Functional Push-up Variations.* Retrieved from https://www.oxygenmag.com/workouts/push-up-prowess

Redl, Alexander (2017). Unsplash. *Photos for everyone.* Retrieved from https://unsplash.com/photos/d3bYmnZ0ank

Hoffman, Matthew (2020). WebMD. *Picture of the Knee.* Retrieved from https://www.webmd.com/pain-management/knee-pain/picture-of-the-knee#1

Fornoni, Tommaso (2017). Unsplash. *Photos for Everyone.* Retrieved from https://unsplash.com/photos/XrzLWellnd0

MacNewton, Curtis (2015). Unsplash. *Photos for Everyone.* Retrieved from https://unsplash.com/photos/5rKPeFcsSTY

Kidport, Reference Library (2012). *Reference Library.* Retrieved from https://www.kidport.com/RefLib/Science/HumanBody/SkeletalSystem/Ankle.htm

Racich, Cole (2015). Advance Physical and Aquatic Therapy. *Lateral Ankle Sprains.* Retrieved from https://advanceaquaticpt.com/lateral-ankle-sprains/

Wikipedia (2020). The Free Encyclopedia. *Ankle.* Retrieved from https://en.wikipedia.org/wiki/Ankle

Krych, Aaron (2011). Hospital for Special Surgery. *Chronic Achilles Tendon Injury*. Retrieved from https://www.hss.edu/conditions_chronic-achilles-tendon-problems-overview.asp

Nascimento, Bruno (2016). Unsplash. *Photos for everyone.* Retrieved from https://unsplash.com/photos/PHIgYUGQPvU

Aldyrkhanov, Artur (2018). Unsplash. *Photos for everyone*. Retrieved from https://unsplash.com/photos/CDpCbaOThwg

Kennaugh, Jonny (2018). Unsplash. *Photos for everyone*. Retrieved from https://unsplash.com/photos/nPOtzvGLYW0

Made in the USA
Columbia, SC
14 June 2020

97852685R00178